The Somatic Internal Family Systems Therapy Workbook

The *The* SOMATIC INTERNAL FAMILY SYSTEMS THERAPY *Workbook*

Embodied Healing Practices *to* Transform Trauma

For therapists, students, clients, and groups

SUSAN McCONNELL

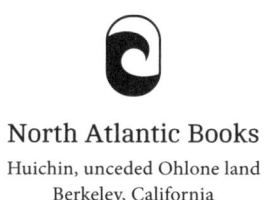

North Atlantic Books
Huichin, unceded Ohlone land
Berkeley, California

North Atlantic Books
Huichin, unceded Ohlone land
2526 Martin Luther King Jr Way
Berkeley, CA 94704 USA
www.northatlanticbooks.com

Cover design by Howie Severson
Book design by Happenstance Type-O-Rama

Printed in Canada

The Somatic Internal Family Systems Therapy Workbook: Embodied Healing Practices to Transform Trauma is sponsored and published by North Atlantic Books, an educational nonprofit based in the unceded Ohlone land Huichin (Berkeley, CA) that collaborates with partners to develop cross-cultural perspectives; nurture holistic views of art, science, the humanities, and healing; and seed personal and global transformation by publishing work on the relationship of body, spirit, and nature.

North Atlantic Books's publications are distributed to the US trade and internationally by Penguin Random House Publisher Services. For further information, visit our website at www.north atlanticbooks.com.

ISBN 979-8-88984-118-0 (pbk.) — ISBN 979-8-88984-119-7 (ebook)

The authorized representative in the EU for product safety and compliance is Eucomply OÜ, Pärnu mnt 139b-14, 11317 Tallinn, Estonia, hello@eucompliancepartner.com, +33757690241.

2 3 4 5 6 7 8 9 MQ 28 27 26 25

Contents

List of Experiential Exercises

Introduction

Including the body story along with the verbal story in therapy illuminates and awakens what has been obscured in darkness.[1]

WITH THESE WORDS, I began my book *Somatic Internal Family Systems Therapy* (2020), and now also this companion workbook, with practical guidelines and exercises to include the body story in therapy. I am Susan McConnell, the founder and developer of Somatic IFS and an IFS Senior Lead Trainer since 1997.

Since the publication of my book at the start of the COVID pandemic, Somatic IFS has expanded beyond my wildest imaginings. Participants of SIFS programs are discovering their bodies to be a source of deep, transformative healing and wisdom. Therapists are realizing that if they only consider thoughts and emotions, they are missing most of the communication. IFS therapists facilitating the relationship between Parts and Self are experiencing how embodying their internal systems with the Somatic IFS practices has illuminated and freed their Embodied Self energy, leading to life-changing transformations. The personal and collective transformations ripple outwards in wider and wider circles, bringing light to the societal forces that have truncated our capacity for embodiment. I am gratified by the commitment and expertise of my growing Somatic IFS staff who continue to contribute in countless ways to the learning and development of Somatic IFS. Many of them have enriched this publication with comments and case examples woven throughout, but especially in chapter 7.

Recently, a Somatic IFS staff member shared that it was her longing to feel more alive, more connected, and more engaged with life that led her to Somatic IFS, where embodying her Self energy has brought her a deeper presence and connection with herself, others, and the world. Responses like this from readers, program participants, and staff have deepened, expanded, and contributed to the evolution of Somatic IFS. They inspire me to bring another Somatic IFS publication with additional practical exercises and guidance for therapists and individuals who, like my staff member, long to feel more alive, connected, and engaged with life.

Who Is This Workbook For?

This Somatic IFS workbook is for those of us longing for fuller embodiment, aliveness, and health. Bridging the chasm between body and mind, this workbook offers practical guidance for therapists, practitioners, and clients as they explore and navigate the intricate intimacies of the bodymind system to address chronic illnesses, addictions, disordered eating, trauma, attachment wounds, sexual and relational issues, and more.

IFS therapists and practitioners will discover the healing potential of incorporating somatic approaches with every step of the IFS Model. Somatic psychotherapists, somatic educators, yoga teachers, bodyworkers, and other physical health professionals will find how integrating the IFS Model can enhance their somatic work with their clients, patients, and students. All those looking for a map to guide them on their journey will be able to explore the mysterious and exquisite territory of their bodymind, and many will realize that the unification of body and mind leads to spirit.

The overarching intention of this workbook is to restore Embodied Self energy to every level of system, from the submolecular to the global. Dispelling the hierarchical binary of mind over body brings to light what has been devalued, exiled, or marginalized. When the burdens locked within the cells and tissues of our individual bodies are freed, the liberated energy ripples out in ever-widening circles. Social activists, spiritual seekers, and all of us who wish to end violence and injustice may find practical information and inspiration to facilitate the kind of profound transformations called for by the current crises. What do you hope to gain from the readings and exercises in this workbook?

❑ To become more embodied.

❑ To find and work with Parts that communicate nonverbally.

❑ To address chronic physical symptoms with the IFS Model.

❑ To become familiar with specific techniques to enrich your clinical practice.

❑ To understand how trauma affects the body and how somatic practices can repair the wounds.

❑ To change the societal norms of objectifying bodies.

❑ Other:

How to Use This Workbook

This Somatic IFS workbook is a companion to *Somatic Internal Family Systems Therapy* (2020). The body of this workbook (chapters 2–6) will cover the five practices of Somatic IFS, and each chapter consists of four main sections:

1. **Purpose of the Practice** introduces the Somatic IFS practice to be explored and experienced and explains the application of this practice towards embodying Self energy in the internal bodymind system.

2. **Individual Application** focuses on individual experiential exercises for anyone interested in exploring their inner system as it is revealed and healed in the body. While primarily focusing on the effects of individual and collective trauma, the exercises are beneficial for other emotional and physical issues. This second section is recommended for therapists, IFS therapists, Somatic IFS therapists, and anyone interested in exploring their bodymind systems to continue developing their own Embodied Self energy. Some of the exercises can be experienced with

a partner or brought to a therapy appointment. The exercises are sequential, but it is not necessary to fully complete each one.

3. **Clinical Application** offers guidance for the therapist to integrate each somatic practice into their clinical interventions. The therapist, having benefited from the explanations and exercises from the second section ("Individual Application"), has become more familiar with their own embodied internal system and has retrained their attentional sensory habits. Many of the exercises in the "Individual Application" section can be used here as is or with some modifications with clients. This third section includes concrete interventions to safely incorporate somatic approaches with every step of the therapeutic process.

4. **Integration** provides an overall reflection of the previous sections of the chapter, incorporating the learnings, takeaways, and next steps needed by Parts to bring completion to this practice while affording a bridge to the next practice.

NOTE ON TERMINOLOGY

In all the exercises in this workbook, the pronoun *it* is used to refer to the Part, unless the Part identifies a gender (he/him, she/her, they/them, etc.). Use the pronoun preferred by the Part. Also, for more guidance with terminology, consider the following chart.

LOWERCASE TERMS	CAPITALIZED TERMS
part refers to any other meaning beyond a subpersonality.	**Part** refers to a subpersonality; in general, it assumes a burdened Part.
Example: She touched the part of her head that was hurting.	Example: She brought her hand to the Part that is using the headache to keep her from having to visit her mother.
self/you refers to the general meaning.	**Self/You** is used to emphasize the person's state of Self energy and not a Part.
Example: I hear that you would rather do this yourself.	Example: Now that your Part knows You are here, and not your critical Part, it is able to receive the Self energy You are sending through your breath.

General Guidelines for Exercises

You may want to record the instructions for the exercises so you can pause your device and follow the steps at your own pace. You can record your responses on your device, a separate notepad, or the space provided after each exercise. You may want to do these exercises with a partner or a therapist while your partner reads the instructions and you can share your experiences.

You will want to find a time and place where you will not be interrupted or distracted, and where you can feel safe and comfortable. Listen to your body and your inner system as you do the exercises to track and assess your level of activation. Although some exercises may be challenging, if you are frequently distracted, or begin to feel spacey, unsafe, or agitated, pause or stop the exercise. Find a way to restore your sense of safety and connection. You may want to have a plan in advance in the event you become uncomfortably activated. As mentioned, there will be safety guidelines throughout the chapters to remind you to attend to your self-care and that of your client.

This workbook is not a substitution for professional help provided by a therapist, psychiatrist, or physician. Some of the information and experiential exercises may not be suitable at this time for you to engage in on your own, or even with a friend or professional. Consult with a trusted and competent professional when appropriate.

Practices and Elements

The five core interdependent practices of Somatic IFS are Somatic Awareness, Conscious Breathing, Radical Resonance, Mindful Movement, and Attuned Touch. These practices are sequential and interdependent, with Somatic Awareness as the foundational practice, and they integrate into every step of the IFS Model to free up burdened Parts so that the internal system can be led by the Embodied Self.

Each practice is associated with a classical element: earth, air, water, and fire. These elements will be included in the chapters, as they assist the exploration of each practice, tie Somatic IFS to collective and ancient healing traditions, and link the human organism—mind, body, and spirit—with the cosmic body made up of these elements. Many ancient cultures have drawn on the healing aspects of these elements to address an array of physical, emotional, and spiritual symptoms. Their accumulated wisdom has contributed to our survival and still informs many of our therapeutic approaches. Although modern science has vastly expanded our understanding of the material world, these elemental forces and sensory experiences link our current modalities to healing legacies from our ancestors and connect us with the larger universe—"the ground below our feet, the air surrounding us, the life-giving waters, the fire that warms our heart and lights our way."[2]

Recommended Reading
To Learn More about the IFS Model

For those interested in a more thorough understanding of the IFS Model, there are many excellent books on the IFS Model available at the bookstore on the website (https://IFS-Institute.com) as well as your favorite independent booksellers. I especially recommend these recent publications:

Seth Kopald, *Self-Led: Living a Connected Life with Yourself and with Others* (Ann Arbor, MI: Exploration Services, 2023).

Richard C. Schwartz, *No Bad Parts: Healing Trauma and Restoring Wholeness with the Internal Family Systems Model* (Boulder, CO: Sounds True, 2021).

Martha Sweezy, *Internal Family Systems Therapy for Shame and Guilt* (New York: Guilford Press, 2023).

Jenna Riemersma, editor, *Altogether Us: Integrating the IFS Model with Key Modalities, Communities, and Friends* (La Vergne, TN: Pivotal Press, 2023).

Frank G. Anderson, *Transcending Trauma: Healing Complex PTSD with Internal Family Systems* (Eau Claire, WI: PESI, 2021).

It will be important for any reader of this workbook to understand the basic assumptions of IFS: multiplicity, the three categories and interrelationships of the subpersonalities (Parts)—managers, firefighters, and exiles—as well as the awareness that everyone has, in addition to Parts, Self energy that can and should lead this internal system of Parts. Along with a cognitive understanding of the IFS Model, the reader will gain the most from this workbook on a somatic approach to IFS if they also have personally experienced either the IFS Model or Somatic IFS.[3]

To Explore Somatic Approaches and Collective Trauma

Manuela Mischke-Reeds, *Somatic Psychotherapy Toolbox: 125 Worksheets and Exercises to Treat Trauma & Stress* (Eau Claire, WI: PESI, 2018).

Susan M. Aposhyan, *Heart Open, Body Awake: Four Steps to Embodied Spirituality* (Boulder, CO: Shambhala, 2021).

Deb Dana and Courtney Rolfe, *Polyvagal Prompts: Finding Connection and Joy through Guided Explorations* (New York: W. W. Norton, 2024).

Gabor Mate, *The Myth of Normal: Trauma, Illness, & Healing in a Toxic Culture* (New York: Avery, 2022).

Thomas Hübl, *Attuned: Practicing Interdependence to Heal Our Trauma—and Our World* (Boulder, CO: Sounds True, 2023).

Notes

1   Susan McConnell, *Somatic Internal Family Systems Therapy: Awareness, Breath, Resonance, Movement and Touch in Practice* (Berkeley, CA: North Atlantic Books, 2020), 1.

2   Susan McConnell, *Somatic Internal Family Systems Therapy*, 49.

3   Susan McConnell, *Somatic Internal Family Systems Therapy*, 17.

1

Somatic IFS

Embodying the Internal Family

The Evolution of Somatic IFS

BECOMING ACQUAINTED WITH DICK SCHWARTZ in the mid-1990s, I was intrigued that his experience with his clients greatly influenced his newly developing IFS Model. I came to understand that all of us have within us an internal family of interacting Parts, which, regardless of their often disastrous impact on our lives, have positive intentions. I then learned that, when the Parts are able to unblend, at the core of every one of us is an inherent source of wisdom, compassion, and clarity known as Self. When our Parts have been wounded, they obscure this Self energy. Therefore, the goal of this empowering, nonpathologizing model is to free the Self and restore the original nature of the Parts so the entire internal family can function harmoniously and collaboratively. Following Dick's example of openly, compassionately, and respectfully listening to his clients, I listened to my clients. I also listened with my body (my eyes, ears, hands) and to my body (my energy, sensations, breath, movements).

Now, over three decades, the experiences of many students and clients have influenced Somatic IFS and have contributed to its evolution. They have come to therapy and SIFS programs to heal the individual traumas and societal burdens that have disconnected them from their bodies. Revisiting their experiences from conception through early childhood has led to their relational, cognitive, social, and physical lives being transformed. They have befriended their protector Parts that use their bodies in numerous ways to do their jobs, containing, controlling, and suppressing the exiles' stories locked in every system of their bodies. As participants and clients have embodied their Parts, the body stories of their formative experiences are witnessed and unburdened, and their Parts' original natures are restored and anchored. IFS therapists have found that when the body stories are welcomed and witnessed by the Embodied Self energy of the therapist and client, the internal systems of both the client and therapist are revised.

How Does Somatic IFS Compare with IFS?

Similarities

Somatic IFS is similar in many ways to IFS. Both stand out from many other psychotherapy models with the assumption of multiplicity rather than a mono-mind perspective. These subpersonalities, or Parts, all have positive intentions. The Parts' original roles become distorted when confronted with extreme situations where they feel overwhelmed and alone. When they can let go of the burdens they acquire from these wounding experiences, they can return to their original valuable qualities. Regarding the Parts as separate from their burdens—as sacred, valuable, interactive beings with respect and compassion—is the remedy for them to release their extreme beliefs, behaviors, and emotions. Another assumption of IFS is that every one of us has a Self that can and should lead the internal system.

At first, it may be the therapist that provides this compassionate presence for the Parts in the client's inner system. As the Parts are able to release their burdened perceptions, beliefs, and emotions, they come to recognize that the client has the same qualities as the therapist. When these Parts restore a trusting relationship with the client's Self, the internal system becomes more harmonious and functional. This relationship is one of the distinguishing and brilliant aspects of the IFS Model. The client's Self is the primary agent of transformation. The therapist facilitates this relationship, and this approach is nonpathologizing, empowering, and *effective.*

I first learned IFS in Dick Schwartz's consultation group. When I shared a challenging session, instead of offering me wise advice, or even explaining this new model he was developing, Dick directed me to listen to my inner system. Finding the Part that was reacting to my client, I brought my Self energy to the Part. It relaxed, and the problem with the client was resolved. In this workbook, every exercise for the therapist begins with the therapist attending to the internal state and restoring their Self energy. This concept is also emphasized in Somatic IFS trainings.

I am still impressed that Dick learned the model primarily from listening to his clients. These concepts are the bedrock of Somatic IFS, along with the techniques for facilitating the steps of the IFS Model.

In Somatic IFS trainings, we use several mnemonic devices that are also used in IFS trainings. To teach the steps of working with Parts, we use words with the letter *F.* The 6 F's, as they are known in the IFS community, are a helpful guide to working with the protective system. They are *find* the Part, *focus* on the Part, *flesh* it out. Then we ask how the client *feels* towards the Part, *befriend* the Part, and ask the Part about its *fears* and address them. These steps are roughly sequential, but the sequence varies from trainer to trainer. Another mnemonic device used by both IFS and Somatic IFS is the 8 C's to describe the qualities of Self energy—compassion, curiosity, clarity, creativity, calm, confidence, courage, and connectedness.

IFS includes the body primarily with two steps of the process: finding the Part and finding the burden of the Part. The client identifies a Part, and the therapist asks, "Where in or around your body do you find this Part?" When the Part's burden is identified, the IFS therapist asks, "Where in your body do you find this burden?"

Differences

Somatic IFS expands on the ways in which IFS includes the body. As the client is sharing verbally, the therapist directs the client to turn their attention to what is happening in their body. If the therapist is aware of gestures, spontaneous touch, or changes in the client's breathing, they may invite the client to notice this body expression to see if it is related to the topic. The client may have Parts that are not ready to shift their attention to the body, and if so, may bring compassionate curiosity to this Part. The Part is found in the body, and the somatic experience of this Part is focused on and fleshed out as the therapist invites the client's curiosity about their embodied Part. The Self of the client is embodied along with all the Parts. The body is included in each step of the process, from developing the Self-to-Part relationship, witnessing the Part's story, unburdening the Part, and inviting and integrating the restored qualities of the Part.

My experience has convinced me that every therapeutic issue can benefit from integrating the somatic aspects of our internal system. So while Somatic IFS does incorporate the five practices with the IFS Model to embody the inner system of Parts and Self, it also includes the body in every step of the process. The sequence of these steps unfolds organically as we track the verbal and nonverbal expressions of the client and their Parts, with the goal of getting to know the Part as it presents itself somatically, and developing a trusting relationship between the Part and the Self of the client.

Although words are important, up to 90 percent of communication is nonverbal, and most of it is outside our awareness. The emphasis on the nonverbal expression of Parts and Self balances out the dominant culture's overemphasis on cognition and verbal expression that has truncated our capacity for our fullest embodied aliveness. Somatic IFS joins many other bodymind approaches as an antidote to those cultural influences.

Very young and traumatized Parts may only communicate nonverbally. Their implicit memories and preverbal attachment trauma are all waiting in the body's tissues and behaviors to be found and healed. That and many other clinical issues can impact bodily as well as mental symptoms and functions.

Somatic IFS assumes that the Self must be embodied for its fullest expression and that the five practices provide a path for this. The 8 C's and other words that describe Self energy have their origin in the body. When the client's Self emerges, the therapist facilitates the client experiencing its embodied state.

Somatic IFS continues to evolve, as does IFS, and I continue to learn from my clients, my students, and my staff. In this way, I have asked my Somatic IFS staff members to share their perspectives on the differences between IFS and Somatic IFS.

Differences with Somatic IFS According to my Staff
SHERRY RUBIN

Although the first F has to do with finding where and how Parts show up and live in the body, it is often a stepping stone in a line heading towards befriending and understanding fears; and then in another line called the "steps of unburdening." Through SIFS, I continually try to cultivate an ongoing, ever-present relationship with the body (mine and the client's), always looping back to sensations, breath, and the five practices.

I always have the linear map within me and return for orientation whenever I am lost. But many Parts, certainly preverbal Parts, do not have the cognitive development to be known through questioning. Without looping back to the body, how everything lives in the body, informs the body, I will miss a lot. I must continually practice fluency in this first language. Although I love IFS, the body is often a step along the way instead of the way. I had dropped using my somatic practices from yoga and yoga nidra in order to learn IFS; when I felt a degree of competence in IFS, I was unsure how to integrate somatic practices. SIFS gave and continues to give me that way within the IFS framework.

What I love about and am always drawn to in SIFS is allowing the somatic wisdom to guide rather than the 6 F's and formal steps of unburdening. I always have those steps in mind. At times, I ask questions from them, but often, the wisdom of the body and Self energy (both the client's and mine) are guiding, not the questions. The steps are always with and within me, as a beloved map.

I have a client who has done no "formal" unburdenings, but her continual and sustained progress with much evidence of healing speaks for itself without the formal steps. When I ask her how the vulnerable ones she worked with last week, last month, or whenever is, she responds with comments like, "She's not hurting anymore, trusts me, and knows I'm here to protect her." When I follow up with a question like, "Does she want anything from you now?" the answer that follows is something like, "She is content where she is and wants me to continue doing what I am doing," or sometimes, "She's fine but she wants me to help the Parts that eat to soothe and cause the weight gain and our physical problems."

MARCELLA COX

Integrating embodiment practices from Susan's model was very supportive to my clinical work, making the home I found with IFS an even warmer and cozier one. Inviting clients to gently return to their bodies and notice what was going on and begin to reinhabit their hearts and bodies deepened my therapeutic work with clients. Being more intentional with embodiment, using Somatic IFS, resulted in me also being more embodied and tracking what was happening internally in my own body. This allowed for a flow of resonance when working with my clients, as well as lending my embodied Self-energy to help my clients slow down to be aware of and compassionately witness the burdened energies in their bodies that longed to be known. Somatic IFS also gave me confidence to invite clients to move, use sound and touch to get to know protectors and exiles, and release burdens from their body.

Another significant shift is that my sessions feel more relational since integrating the five practices of Somatic IFS into my clinical work. I attribute this to having greater embodied Self energy, and actually feeling more what my clients are sharing with me. I am now experiencing the 8 C's of Self energy as relational energies—feeling the qualities of curiosity, the compassion, the connectedness in my body—and my clients' systems also sense more of my Self energy, which is inherently relational.

I also attribute this to the practice of Radical Resonance, which allows my heart, body, and right brain to attune to the subtle energies of my clients' Parts and be in embodied flow with my client's system while being in my own Self energy. My clients have shared that they feel really felt by me in our sessions. I believe that clients come for Somatic IFS but stay for the therapeutic relationship enhanced by the practice of Radical Resonance.

DARIO MARTINEZ

Somatic IFS invites us to expand our conceptualization of what it means to "listen." Processing spoken language is one form of listening, but we can also listen through feelings, sensations, vibrations, and energy.

These forms of listening can be vitally important in therapy because a person's unspoken communication often describes their current situation much more accurately and with greater precision than spoken words. My client endorsed this idea at the end of our session by thanking me for helping her to understand what was *actually* happening for her—instead of what she *thought* was happening for her.

As babies, we don't have words to communicate our needs to our caregivers. Human beings are natural experts at using implicit communication to get our needs met. As we get older, our rational "thinking" Parts begin to dominate—and implicit forms of communication become largely unconscious and ultimately ignored. Through the practices of Somatic IFS, we're able to reclaim our ability to respond effectively to each other's implicit primal messages. We're able to *see* each other in ways that many of us have not experienced since we were babies. This can feel like a kind of *homecoming* for many of our clients.

LESLEY HARTMAN

I find SIFS and IFS look and feel *very* different, even though I experience SIFS as following the same steps as IFS. For me, in SIFS, the steps of the model emerge more from the client and my responses are more resonant and attuned to the client's Parts. I experience the steps of the model in SIFS as driven less from me as the therapist than in standard IFS. The pacing is slower, and the steps are achieved in a more scaffolded manner that is more attuned to the client's system.

I also find less need to verbalize all the steps; so they are happening, but not always as a result of my line of questioning. There is a wider range of communication options for Parts, and for me, that helps my more scientific-analytical psychologist Parts to relax into the wider ocean of Self clarity without the need to internally case conceptualize or ask the clients' Parts to constantly translate from nonverbal-somatic to verbal. I have found this really helpful myself to stay Self-led, as I have always had strong intuitive knowing, which certain psychologist Parts would doubt or question or require evidence for (to a degree that would take me outside the circle of connection with the client). I also notice that my clients' less verbal Parts open up more, and that their Self-like, analytical, and pleaser Parts that want to give the right answers get engaged less often in SIFS.

It took a long time for my more analytical psychologist Parts to step back and trust my more intuitive Self in therapy. Now it feels hard to undo my SIFS learning, as I try to simply follow the line of questioning that will demonstrate my knowledge of the IFS model. I feel more robotic, more verbal and intellectual, less attuned, and like I am robbing myself of a whole tool kit that helps me connect more deeply with Self and with the clients' Parts. It feels to my own less verbal and more intuitive Parts like regression to a time when their ways of knowing were sidelined. From this, I gather that in my system, some Parts experience IFS as privileging more verbal ways of communicating and of knowing, ways that in my life have been linked to dominant (male) culture.

I have also noticed that IFS questioning can be taken as an invitation for response from strong intellectual-analytical or Self-like Parts in my clients, and that this can interrupt the Self-to-Part healing process. In SIFS, in contrast, these Parts are more able to relax back. It feels like in SIFS there is an unsaid communication that whatever pace or manner in which the Parts communicate is OK. There is no rush. Inherent in a more verbal questioning approach is a subtle pressure for Parts to respond in that same way. Perhaps that comes from my Parts rather than from the process itself. I don't know!

Embodying the Internal Family
Parts and the Body

Protector Parts use the body to do their jobs, either proactively (managers) or reactively (firefighters). Their job is to lock our vulnerable Parts away where they cannot flood our systems. The tragic side effect of their protection is that the exiled Parts cannot heal. The protectors see their jobs as crucial to our survival and will devotedly and strategically use whatever is at hand to keep the system from perceived harm, including the body's structures, behaviors, and energies. Weight gain or loss, addictive behaviors, disordered eating, self-harming behaviors, acute or chronic illness, even accidents—all and more may be orchestrated by protector Parts.

> Any healthy or necessary behavior—exercise, eating, sleeping, sex, touch, breathing, even altruistic caring for others—can be enlisted by the Part to protect itself, other Parts, or the internal system. Like good investors, they can diversify. Like football players, they are strategic. They can block, push, run, tackle, counter, and pass. They are creative. They know how to build effective walls to keep out and to imprison. They can turn the body into a fortress by blocking or buttressing energies at the joints, in the diaphragms, and in the lower back. They get hold of our internal pharmaceuticals. They send hormones to affect heart and breath rates. They do what they have to do to keep the individual from getting hurt or being overwhelmed by past hurts. The therapist keeps in mind that any of these physical signs may indicate the behavior of a protector Part.[1]

The 6 F's guide the process of bringing the presence of Self energy to the protectors. As they come to trust the Self, the more vulnerable Parts they have been diligently protecting are free to emerge.

Exiles use the body to tell their stories. These vulnerable Parts are often younger than protector Parts. Their hurtful experiences, needs, shame, and pain are suppressed and, well, exiled. Their stories and burdens are found everywhere in the body, in every system, cell, and part of the cell. These Parts inhabit the body and have bodies of their own that may be different from the individual's body. For example, a client may report that their young Part has collapsed, yet they are sitting upright. Or the client's body may collapse in the chair.

Trauma shatters the cohesive verbal and nonverbal narrative of their story. Traumatized Parts may have been threatened if they tell the verbal story. Parts may have suppressed their bodily memories from the fear that the sensations will overwhelm the system. The somatic aspects of the story may be disturbing, fragmented, and intrusive physical symptoms, and this may be all that can be accessed of their painful story.

Witnessing the Body Story and Releasing Burdens Frozen in the Body

> With these vulnerable exile Parts, even more than with the protectors, the Somatic IFS therapist relies on nonverbal communication. Often their wounds from relational trauma occurred long before they had the capacity to consciously remember, long before they had the words to tell their stories. If these wounds occurred any time from conception through the first four or five years of life, the client's story of the pain or disruption will be told through the body's sensations and movements and disruptions in sensation and movement.[2]

Self and the Body

The 8 C's (compassion, curiosity, clarity, creativity, calm, confidence, courage, and connectedness) and other words that describe the qualities of Self can find their expression in body sensations, breath, movement, and touch. Self energy, resonating with Parts and conveying these qualities to Parts nonverbally, creates a strong, resilient, safe, and intimate bond. Therapists can convey Self energy through their body with a relaxed, aligned, centered posture; eye contact; a relaxed, warm facial expression; a slow, full breath; and a warm, respectful touch.

The Therapist and Somatic IFS

The first step of all the exercises in this workbook is for the therapist to establish their own Self energy. Although techniques are an important part of an IFS training, I never forgot the lesson from Dick Schwartz that the therapist's Self energy trumps any technique. In the first training where I assisted Dick, my manager Parts worked hard to stay one step ahead of the students. Eventually, I developed enough confidence that my managers could step aside, freeing up my Self presence with clients and students. Over the years, I have identified many subtle protectors that are called in IFS "Self-like Parts." These manager Parts are often our older, parentified child Parts that do not yet know or trust our Self. As they come to trust my compassionate awareness and appreciation of their intention—and how long and hard they have carried the huge burden of responsibility—they make space for more of my Embodied Self energy to lead.

Just as an IFS therapist prioritizes their own Self energy over techniques and interventions to assist the client's internal world, a Somatic IFS therapist attends to their internal state to access their Embodied Self energy. They tune into their inner world and become adept at reading their body's signals to differentiate Parts from Self. They have learned how to quickly and effectively reassure their Parts that their Self can lead the way. Somatic IFS therapists have regular practices that cultivate their Self energy and provide "first aid" techniques for those times before or during a session when Parts believe they need to take over the therapist's role. Each therapist finds what works best for them to restore their Self energy. The upcoming exercises are an opportunity to experience whether the somatic practices can be helpful to your inner system when a Part takes over your therapist role.

EXPERIENTIAL EXERCISE
THE SOMATIC IFS THERAPIST'S SELF-TO-PART RELATIONSHIP

1. When you feel ready, turn your full attention inwards to notice the state of your internal system—Parts and Self. What are the indicators of a Part? Of Self energy?

2. If you only find Self energy, enjoy it! Send it out to the wider world.

3. If you find a Part taking over your system, let's discover what helps your Part so you can more fully feel your Embodied Self energy. Acknowledge and accept the Part with a friendly, internal nod. Be curious about what this Part might need from You in order to relax and trust You to be in the therapist's chair.

4. Bring your awareness to the sensations of your feet and your seat as they connect with the floor and the chair, making adjustments to how you are sitting. Is this helpful?

5. Bring your awareness to your breathing, again making any changes with how you are sitting so your breathing is supported. Breathe in, breathe out longer, for at least five breaths.

6. Scan your body for places of tension or places that are more difficult to feel. Try moving or touching these places.

7. Check in with the Part. If the Part needs more, continue with the next exercise. Or, in the next exercise, you can choose to work with a familiar therapist Part that sometimes obscures your Self energy.

EXPERIENTIAL EXERCISE
WORKING SOMATICALLY WITH THE FIRST 4 F'S

1. **Find a Part:** How does this Part first show itself to you—thoughts, words, images, emotions, beliefs, behaviors, impulses to move, physical sensations?

2. **Focus on the Part:** Keep your focused, open attention on the ways this Part first shows up for several moments. Notice what unfolds. Follow your curiosity about what the Part is letting you know. If another Part distracts you, gently bring your attention back to the Part.

3. Flesh out the Part:

If the somatic aspect of the Part emerges spontaneously, bring your awareness to the sensations—the size, texture, weight—anything else you are curious about. If the Part shows up first as thoughts, words, visual images, or memory, invite the somatic aspect of the Part.

- What happens in your body as you hear or speak these words from your Part?
- What does the Part believe about itself, you, others, or the world? How does your body express this belief?
- What does this Part do or cause other Parts to do?
- Facilitate the relationship between Self and Part:

4. How do you feel towards this Part?

If you feel openness, curiosity, or acceptance (indicating Self energy), tune in to this state where you find it in your body. Communicate this Self energy to the Part and let these sensations flow towards this Part.

- Is this Part aware of your Self presence? How does this Part feel towards You (your Self)? What happens in your body as this Part begins to connect with and trust You?
- Thank the Part for trusting you. Let it know you will come back to it later to find out more about what it needs from you.
- If instead of feeling open and accepting, you feel critical, annoyed, afraid, or any other feeling or attitude, this indicates a second Part. Can this Part step aside, or does it need your attention first?
- How do you feel towards this second Part?
- Follow the above prompts to work with this second Part.
- When this second Part's needs have been met, proceed to bring your Self energy back to Part 1 and form a connection with it from Self.

EXPERIENTIAL EXERCISE
BRINGING SELF TO SELF-LIKE MANAGER PARTS

1. Invite one of your hardworking manager Parts to come forward. Bring your compassionate, curious presence to it.

2. Ask the Part to show you how it adopts the qualities, or one of the qualities, of Embodied Self energy: clarity, curiosity, courage, compassion, confidence, creativity, calmness, connectedness.

3. Can you tell the difference between when this quality is expressed by this Part and when it is expressed by your Self?

4. Bring any of the Somatic IFS practices and interventions you have developed to establish and deepen a Self-to-Part relationship with this Part. There may need to be a relational repair with this Part if it has experienced a lack of respect and appreciation from other Parts in your system.

5. Ask this Part what it will need going forward to let go of its burdens and to grow to trust You.

With the exercises above, you have experienced how Parts can show up in your body, and you have brought Embodied Self energy to your Parts. The next exercise offers you an opportunity to identify your therapist Parts that come up in general or with a specific client so that your Parts will be more willing to trust your Self to be in the therapist chair. You may want to practice this exercise with a partner sitting in the client's chair who can stand in for the client who activates your Parts.

EXPERIENTIAL EXERCISE
WHICH CHAIR TO SIT ON?

1. Arrange two chairs next to each other. One is the Self-led therapist chair, and the other the Part-led therapist chair. Sit in the Self chair.

2. Name some situations with clients that tend to activate your Parts.

3. Choose one to focus on.

4. Imagine and describe this situation with all your senses.

5. What Parts arise? How do they make their presence known to you?

6. Choose one Part to focus on.

7. Sit in the Part-led therapist chair, imagining your client before you. Invite your Part to become embodied. Notice how this Part shows up in your body.

8. Remaining sitting in the Part-led chair, how do you feel towards the client?

9. Imagine how the scene plays out as you interact with the client with this Part in the lead during the session.

10. Sit in the Self-led therapist chair, imagining your client before you. Take some time to fully embody Self energy. How does Self energy show up in your body?

11. Remaining sitting in the Self-led therapist chair, notice how you feel towards the client. Imagine how the scene plays out as you interact with the client from your Embodied Self energy.

12. Move the Part-led therapist chair in front of you and invite your Part to sit there. Bring your attention to the Part sitting in the Part-led therapist chair. How do you feel towards this Part? What does it want you to know about it?

13. What does this Part need from you to trust You to be in the Self-led therapist chair with this situation?

The Somatic IFS Therapist and the Client

One of the first steps in the IFS Model as well as in Somatic IFS is to consider if the client's external situation will support transformative work. This includes understanding the client's home life, work life, and relational life for the level of safety and resources. It also includes the client's response to the physical therapeutic environment, and the therapist can make accommodations to create a safe, potentially healing environment.

THERAPIST ASSESSES THE EXTERNAL SITUATION FOR THE CLIENT

- In person: How is the distance between the therapist and client? Are there any external triggers in the room or office? If possible, remove them.

- Virtual: Does a virtual long-distance therapeutic relationship provide adequate connection for the needs of the client's system? Does the client prefer online or phone? How is the lighting, audio, distance (size), background?

THERAPIST ASSESSES THE INTERNAL STATE OF THE CLIENT IN THE PRESENT MOMENT

- The therapist notes their client's physical state (tired, hungry, frightened), movement (agitated, collapsed, held), posture, stance, eyes, face, and voice (pitch, volume, flowing, or hesitant).

- The therapist holds all this data with curiosity and compassion, without assumptions or interpretations.

Difficulties in therapy can often be traced to unclear agreements about the objective of therapy, the hoped-for outcomes, and the issues to be addressed in therapy. Therefore, early in the relationship, the therapist and client will come to an agreement, checking with their Parts to see if there is a common agreement. This "contract" is a mutual process and may need to be revisited frequently, both because it may change and because considering the initial agreement can reset the direction of the process.

THERAPIST AND CLIENT ESTABLISH AN INITIAL CONTRACT

- The client states the issue or Parts they want to work with and the anticipated outcome.

- The therapist asks the client what they notice in their body as they state what they want to address in therapy. The therapist tracks the client's nonverbal communication for any inconsistencies with their verbal statement.

- The therapist listens internally to any Parts with concerns or objections regarding the client's stated issue.

- Once a mutual agreement has been reached, the therapist and client may discuss the steps of the process towards this outcome.

- The therapist asks the client to go inside to find any Parts with concerns about working with this issue. The therapist clarifies and names the protector Parts.

- The therapist asks for an agreement to first work with any protector Parts related to the client's issue.

Having established their Embodied Self energy, assessed the external situation, and formed a mutual agreement with their client about what to work on and how to work together, the therapist's next step is to help the client turn their attention inwards. Any of the Somatic IFS practices can be useful to explore their internal system with an open, curious attitude. When a Part shows up as thoughts, words, memory, images, or emotions, the following exercise can be a guide to include the somatic aspect of the Part.

EXPERIENTIAL EXERCISE
FINDING A PART

1. Include the somatic aspect of the Part if the Part first presents otherwise:

   - As you hear those words, feel that emotion, see that image, etc., what do you notice is happening in your body?

   - Where in your body do those thoughts and emotions reside?

   - How does your body express this belief?

   - Would the Part like to show us this behavior with a movement?

The therapist applies the process they used to work with their own Parts in the exercise "Working Somatically with the First 4 F's" to *find, focus, flesh out,* and *facilitate the relationship* (sometimes referred to as *befriending*) with the protector Part that the client has identified. The client's Part will feel the presence of the therapist's Self and possibly also their own Self and will feel known in its entirety—verbally and nonverbally. These first four steps lead naturally to the next steps, which also have words with the letter F: *finding out* what the Part wants you to know, and addressing the Part's *fears.*

PARTS' NONVERBAL COMMUNICATION

For many clients, awareness of the body is the only available channel for their Parts and their stories to be known. For other Parts, words may accompany the body story, like subtitles in a foreign film. The body, sculpted by history, provides the third dimension to the oral account. If the physical aspect of the Part is not evident, if instead the Part first shows itself to us as a thought, image, or emotion, we invite the Part to be known in its fleshed-out fullness. To miss the body story of the Part is to be missing most of the show.[3]

Our clients may have a coherent verbal narrative of their personal histories that they explicitly remember, but what of their histories before they had language? What of the events of their lives that have been exiled, suppressed, and erased from their conscious memories? These stories are waiting to be told through sensations and movement impulses. The thwarted experiences, overwhelming traumas, or faulty attachments that bring our client to seek therapy are revealed before that client even opens their mouth to speak. The same can be said for ourselves.

Parts that first emerge with thoughts, feelings, images, and words can be known more fully as the nonverbal aspects are invited. This topic will be covered further in chapter 2; however, I want to first address it here since nonverbal communication applies to all the practices, not only Somatic Awareness. Additionally, the following exercise invites your curiosity to get to know the nonverbal expression of a Part.

EXPERIENTIAL EXERCISE
SHIFTING FROM VERBAL TO NONVERBAL EXPRESSION

1. Invite a Part that shows up primarily verbally. It might speak to you or let you know how it is feeling, what it is thinking, what it believes.

2. Let the Part know you hear it, that you understand what it is telling you. Notice what happens with the Part.

3. Ask the Part if it would be willing to tune in to what is happening in the body as it shares these thoughts with you. The Part itself may have a bodily experience, or you may notice some place in your body that is associated with the Part's thoughts or emotions. You may notice a physical sensation, an energetic shift, a movement or impulse to move, a change in your breath. The Part itself may have a movement or behavior it expresses. If so, stay with the nonverbal aspect that the Part is sharing with you and let it know you are hearing and holding all it is telling you

4. Record any differences, difficulties, benefits of including the nonverbal aspects of this Part.

Integration

1. What differences between Somatic IFS and IFS intrigued you?

_____

_____

_____

2. Did you find protector Parts that use your body to do their jobs? What are their jobs, and how do they use your body?

_____

_____

_____

3. Are you aware of any vulnerable Parts that use your body to tell their story?

_____

_____

_____

4. Which qualities of Self energy did you find in your bodily sensations or behaviors?

_____

_____

_____

5. Are there any Parts you discovered that need more attention from You, or from the support of another person in addition? What can you promise the Part?

_____

_____

_____

6. Did you find a Part that only communicates or expresses itself nonverbally?

_____

_____

_____

7. If you are a therapist, what would you say is the importance of starting with ourselves as therapists and health care professionals?

_____

_____

_____

8. As a therapist, have you found that a clear contract at the beginning and revisited during the course of therapy has been helpful? Have you found that some Parts have not "bought in"?

_____

_____

_____

9. What therapist Parts did you discover that you would like to continue to address?

_____

_____

_____

10. What difficulties do you experience helping your client shift their attention inwards, or to be open to listening to their bodies?

_____

_____

_____

11. What questions do you have about a somatic approach to therapy, or to IFS therapy, that you hope will be answered in future chapters?

_____

_____

_____

Notes

1 Susan McConnell, *Somatic Internal Family Systems Therapy,* 31.

2 Susan McConnell, *Somatic Internal Family Systems Therapy,* 35.

3 Susan McConnell, *Somatic Internal Family Systems Therapy,* 64.

2

Somatic Awareness

Purpose of Somatic Awareness

SOMATIC AWARENESS, AS THE FIRST of the five Somatic IFS practices, lays the framework for the practices of Conscious Breathing, Radical Resonance, Mindful Movement, and Attuned Touch. All of these practices are integrated with the IFS Model to restore Embodied Self energy.

Attending to our body sensations, we find Parts that use our body sensations to perform their roles and send messages, be they subtle or profound. That is to say, the Parts feel our connection and use the body as their primary vehicle for communication. Grounded in our bodily experience, unfolding moment by moment, the inherent wisdom embedded in our body becomes available to us.

The adjective *somatic* in Somatic Awareness sets the stage by referring to the subjective rather than objective experience of our bodies. We tend to use the left hemisphere of our brains and manager Parts that are good at evaluation, assessment, measuring, and fixing. Plus, an objective view is quantitative, external. All of this is valuable. As for a subjective focus, it involves the right hemisphere of the brain and yields different information and Parts. It is qualitative and internal. Therefore, we might think that objective information is more factual and true, but there are different truths that arise with a subjective experience. These truths allow us to access our internal experiences.

EXPERIENTIAL EXERCISE
OBJECTIVE AND SUBJECTIVE AWARENESS OF THE BODY

1. Focus on your hand from an objective point of view. Notice visually the size, shape, veins, skin, nails, palm, and back of your hand. Move your hand to notice the strength or flexibility of your hands and fingers. What Parts get engaged in objectively viewing your hand?

2. Focus on your other hand to explore the difference of a subjective experience of your hand. You might want to close your eyes so you aren't distracted visually.

3. Bring your awareness as fully as possible to the sensations in your hand. Take several minutes to notice sensations on the skin, the muscles, bones, circulation, the energy flow, temperature, weight, pulsations, impulses to move—any sensations that draw your attention.

4. Shift from being aware of these sensations to centering your attention *within* these sensations. There may just be sensations, or you may find words that label or describe the sensations.

5. How do you feel towards this hand?

6. Stay focused on your hand for as long as you desire. Do any images of your hand come to you?

7. Now compare this hand with your other hand that you viewed objectively. What differences between the hands do you notice?

8. As you open your eyes and complete this exercise, you might journal about the difference between an objective and subjective experience of your hand, or show it in a drawing.

Awareness of our subjective experience of our bodies is a superpower. It awakens and enlivens our entire bodymind systems. It is like love. It informs, amplifies, and deepens every step of the IFS Model, leading to the state of Embodied Self. We bring a focused, open attention to body sensations and lack of sensation as they unfold moment by moment, revealing the body story of the Part. Awareness is central to any healing process. With Somatic IFS, as we cultivate our capacity for awareness of our body with the practice of Somatic Awareness, we release burdens from an objectifying world from where they were frozen in the body, restoring our vibrancy, connection, grace, and power. We again inhabit our body. We are *being* a body rather than *having* a body.

Many of our life experiences have blunted our innate capacity for awareness. Individual and collective traumas are embedded in all the tissues of our bodies, stripping us of our birthright to be fully embodied. Hurtful messages and experiences from our individual lives and societal messages result in protectors that hate, fear, avoid, or ignore our bodies. When we have the intention to bring more attention to our bodies, there may be a cast of internal characters waiting in the wings to take center stage. Typically, our bodies get our attention when there is something wrong. A concerned protective Part may take over to try to fix the problem or find someone who can. Other Parts put the body's needs as a low priority. Just as an IFS session first invites and welcomes the protector Parts, we begin in Somatic IFS with those protector Parts that believe their job is to block our awareness.

We can invite these Parts to take a bow, thank them for the roles they have played so well in the past, and see if they may want to sit in the front row of the audience to find out what happens next. The exercise below will help us to notice our body sensations and any Parts with concerns about body awareness.

SAFETY GUIDELINES

If you begin to feel overwhelmed, activated, or dissociated as you do the exercises in this chapter, take a pause to bring your attention to the safety in the present moment.

Listen to the activated Parts. When they are ready, and you feel grounded, curious, and calm, you can come back to the exercise.

EXPERIENTIAL EXERCISE

TUNING INTO THE BODY

Find a comfortable place to sit or lie down to focus on your body for about five minutes. Be prepared to record what you notice in a voice recording or a notepad.

1. Bring awareness to your body. You might begin by scanning from top to bottom, or just notice what draws your attention.

2. Are there words that describe your present body sensations?

3. Notice what places ask for your attention. Where? Is it one place or many?

4. Choose one to focus on. How does this place feel to you?

5. Name the sensations you are aware of now. The sensations may change as you notice them.

6. Do any Parts come up that distract you? If so, find out their concerns and see what they need to allow you to bring your focus back to the sensation for another couple of minutes.

7. As you stay with the sensation, how are you feeling towards it?

8. Do you sense any feelings or thoughts that seem connected to the sensation? If so, does it lead to a Part of you that may be connected with this sensation?

9. If you find a Part connected with this sensation, let it know you are listening to it and open to whatever it wants you to know.

10. Are there any changes in this sensation at the end of the five minutes?

11. Scan your body one more time to notice any other changes in your body.

Individual Application of Somatic Awareness
When Our Parts Fear Somatic Awareness

There are numerous reasons why our Parts fear, block, or hesitate to engage in noticing our bodies. Early childhood traumas, later traumas, current or historical chronic pain and illnesses, ancestral legacies, and painful past experiences with physical health providers are only a few that have resulted in many of us distrusting, disliking, blaming, avoiding, and punishing our bodies.

Some of our Parts' beliefs and fears might be outmoded, while others might be quite accurate, sensing that the outer or inner environment will not support a change in our inner system. Below are some concerns about awareness of the body that might arise from our Parts. Check any belief or fear that you find your Parts carry:

- ❑ They fear being overwhelmed by painful or troubling symptoms from an illness.
- ❑ They fear uncovering traumatic burdens and being overwhelmed by sensory flashbacks.
- ❑ They have successful strategies of avoiding and suppressing the body story, such as unleashing our stash of psychopharmaceuticals, and see no good reason to stop doing it.
- ❑ They have learned to distrust and dislike our bodies.
- ❑ They have absorbed societal burdens that objectify our bodies.
- ❑ They are critical of our bodies—blame them, punish them.
- ❑ They want to fix or improve our bodies or our bodily functions.
- ❑ They are polarized with a Part that is wanting, even desperate for, attention paid to the body.
- ❑ They don't trust the body as a source of wisdom or information, but rather as a source of pain or shame.
- ❑ They fear they won't do it right.
- ❑ They have not experienced the body to be a place of safety or pleasure.
- ❑ They believe that focusing on the body will worsen their mental or physical symptoms.
- ❑ They have a habit of avoiding or ignoring the body.
- ❑ Other:

_____

It is common for several opposing Parts to emerge when we try something new. One Part wants to do the exercise. Another Part feels reluctant. Another Part tries to get rid of the reluctant Part, causing it to dig in its heels. Appreciation and respect from Self disarms the reluctant protector. The protector can watch from the wings as we bring awareness to our bodily structures, sensations, and symptoms, and it may come to trust that awareness can be a good thing.

EXPERIENTIAL EXERCISE
ADDRESSING THE PROTECTOR PART'S FEARS

1. Which fear do you want to focus on?

2. How do you feel towards this Part that has some fear about focusing on your body?

3. If your answer is that you want this Part to be different, that indicates another Part. Let this second Part know you want to bring an attitude of acceptance and curiosity to the protector Part that holds fears in the hopes that it can be different. Is this second Part willing to trust You?

4. If so, bring a compassionate, curious presence to the protector Part. Ask your Part if it would share more about its fears or beliefs about you bringing awareness to your body.

5. Ask the Part when it took on this job of protecting you.

6. Let the Part know you understand it. You appreciate that it wants you to be safe, and you want that too. Reassure the Part that you won't override it or try to trick it. How does this Part respond?

7. What does the Part need in order to trust that things could be different now?

The trauma stored in our bodies—which can come in the form of tension, numbness, collapsed posture, chronic illness—awaits the power of our compassionate awareness. We bring compassionate awareness to body sensations and lack of sensation in order to free Parts of their burdens and restore Embodied Self energy. Awareness of the body awakens our inherent but often obstructed body awareness.

CULTURAL BURDENS

Our family, community, ethnicity, and subcultures shape our attitudes and behaviors towards our bodies. Standards of beauty and the ways we do appreciate and care for our bodies may stem from years of tradition and deeply held beliefs. While in some respects, some of us have enough reason to bring gratitude to members of our family, community, or ancestral lines for the ways they have helped us regard our body positively, there are still many cultural beliefs that influence our internal systems to hold a negative view of our bodies.

Several hundred years of Western Eurocentric paradigms have separated mind and body, devaluing and objectifying the body. Value is attributed to some bodies, such as those that are White, male, young, slim, nondisabled, straight, and cisgender, while other bodies are devalued, such as those that are Black, Brown, female, very young or old, large, disabled, and LGBTQ+. Societal institutions—family, community, educational, religious, media and entertainment, economic, health care—implicitly and explicitly convey these beliefs that we absorb collectively and individually. More recently, social media, advertising, and technology have falsely promoted unrealistic and unattainable body images. The burdens we have absorbed from negative societal messages about our bodies have, as mentioned, caused our Parts to fear, avoid, or even hate our bodies.

Bringing a compassionate awareness to the burdened Parts is the first step to ending the criticism, hatred, disconnection, objectification, and neglect of our bodies. A somatic approach to knowing our bodies is the remedy for objectification.

EXPERIENTIAL EXERCISE
UNCOVERING CULTURAL BURDENS

1. Name the ways your body, or particular aspects of your body, have been valued and rewarded.

2. When and how did you become aware of these cultural beliefs?

3. How has this cultural valuation affected your body, emotions, beliefs, and behaviors?

4. Name the ways your body, or particular aspects of your body, have been devalued, criticized, or exiled.

5. When and how did you become aware of these cultural beliefs?

6. How have these cultural burdens affected your body, emotions, beliefs, and behaviors?

7. How do you feel today towards these aspects of your body? Take some time to bring your compassionate presence to these Parts and places in your body that have not been valued and accepted.

The power of a deep, sustained, compassionate awareness can melt the protector Parts, uncovering the vulnerable Parts they have been dedicated to protecting. These exiled Parts who have been hidden in fear and shame long to be known, to have their stories heard. Their stories may not be able to be told verbally. Sensation is often the first word of the body story waiting to be heard, witnessed, and released. Somatic Awareness gives them the language of sensation that can be witnessed and resonated with, bringing forth a new story of safety, freedom, and full aliveness.

The following exercise can guide you to bring awareness to your body. Be prepared to record what you notice with a voice recording, a notepad, or the space provided after the exercise. If Parts distract you during this exercise, tend to the Part and gently bring your attention back to your body.

EXPERIENTIAL EXERCISE
NOTICING YOUR BODY SENSATIONS

1. Find a comfortable place to sit or lie down to focus on your body for several minutes with the intention to notice your sensations.

2. Check with the protector Parts you found earlier to see if they are willing to let you bring your awareness to your body. If they have any concerns, find out what they need.

3. Check for any other Parts—Parts that want to change or fix, or that analyze, judge, or distract. Ask them if they can relax and trust your Self to notice your body sensations for a few minutes.

4. You may choose to begin by tuning into your body and notice what sensations first show up. Or you may choose to direct your awareness, scanning your entire body or focusing on a particular part of your body, like your skin, muscles, bones, or organs.

5. What sensations do you notice?

6. Are there some places in your body that are more difficult to feel?

7. Choose one sensation to focus on for a few minutes.

8. How are you feeling towards this sensation?

9. Your answer lets you know if there is a Part that is aware rather than your Self. If so, this Part might be willing to step back and bring your curiosity, acceptance, and openness to this sensation.

10. Notice what happens with the sensation as You stay with it. How is it the same? How does it change?

11. As you stay with this sensation, are there emotions, thoughts, or images that seem to be associated with the sensation?

12. If so, it may be that this sensation is the first "word" of a Part that wants your attention. Let the Part know that You are with it. You might get a sense if the Part is aware of You. Be open to anything it wants You to know.

13. As you come to completion, has the sensation changed? In what ways is it the same, and in what ways is it different?

_____

_____

_____

Nonverbal to Verbal Translation

The next step after noticing our sensations is to name them. Naming our nonverbal experience is an important part of the process of Somatic IFS, as it integrates the verbal and nonverbal functions of our brain—the left (verbal language) and right (body and emotion) hemispheres. Naming our nonverbal experiences is like learning a new language. Often it is not easy to differentiate between a sensation, emotion, or thought when describing our experience. Sometimes the distinction is blurry. It might not even be important. But it is always useful to value both functions of our brains.

For example, the word *irritated* can describe a bodily sensation or an emotional state. As we stay curious about how we physically experience the emotional state of irritation, we may find our jaw clenched, our upper body tensely held, our fingers contracted, and our lower body numb. We may notice our entire skin is sensitive, and we may feel the impulse to recoil from physical contact. If instead we stop at the emotional state, often a parade of thoughts marches in that convinces us of their validity: "That person is rude and inconsiderate." "I am too sensitive." "I never should have come here." "Maybe I am coming down with something." Staying with the sensations can intercept the compelling narrative of our protectors that blame, project, distract, and otherwise try to soothe us from this irritation. When these thoughts fade into the background, we bring our full attention to the sensations. We find the Part amid these sensations and bring to it our compassionate presence.

SOME OF THE WORDS WE USE TO NAME SENSATIONS

tense	held	numb	flowing	trembling	shaky	moving
cold	warm	heavy	light	tight	loose	calm
burning	aching	dense	still	relaxed	alive	restless
itchy	prickly	blocked	swirling	stuck	full	empty
collapsed	open	expanded	condensed	agitated	irritated	solid

EXPERIENTIAL EXERCISE
DEVELOPING OUR ABILITY TO NAME SENSATIONS

1. There are many words that we use to describe our current states that don't specifically describe a physical experience. *Confused, disoriented, left out, lonely, joyous, excited, anxious, lost, embarrassed, annoyed,* and *grateful* are just a few of them.

2. Remember a time you felt one of these ways. Stay with the experience. Embody it. Notice how it shows up in your body, and find some words to describe the physical sensations.

3. Identify an emotional state you are aware of feeling in this moment.

4. Are there thoughts and beliefs that go along with how you are feeling?

5. Come back to the emotion and invite it to show itself to you. Invite it to be embodied, even exaggerated. Where do you feel that in your body?

6. Notice the sensation or sensations. Find a word or words that best describe this state. Bring your acceptance and open presence to this Part. Let your Part know you are aware of it, its emotion, and how it shows up in your body.

Earth Element

When I consciously connect with the earth, my young Parts show me how I used to frequently escape to the nearby woods. Climbing trees, watching birds flit from branch to branch, and observing insects crawl over mounds of fallen leaves brought me peace and connection to something larger than my life, as it does today. Sometimes it brings sadness and guilt as I remember those who walked this land before my ancestors violently took it from them, and how the earth and its inhabitants have been exploited.

Earth has been considered our Mother in countless cultures, through the millennia. She has given us everything we need for life—shelter, plants for food, medicine, beauty, and fellow animals that fly, swim, crawl, and walk on the earth. IFS recognizes that Self energy is not limited to humans; it also abides in other animate beings as well as inanimate beings. That energy is more available to us for our well-being than we typically recognize. In the second chapter of *Somatic Internal Family Systems Therapy,* I mention some ways the practice of Somatic Awareness draws on our connection to Mother Earth.

> We bring our awareness to the floor or the chair below us and connect with the earth, allowing our energies to ground and center. We appreciate how the earth has abundantly supported us, how we have planted seeds and harvested during our lifetimes. We walk in the footsteps of so many who have walked the earth before us. We are grounded and supported every step of the way. The earth knows the rhythms and cycles of change, the mountainous heights and the deep darkness of caves. Connecting again and again to the earth, we develop a dependable anchor in the face of tumultuous emotional energies. Perhaps we can assist *ourselves and our clients* to find safety and support from the earth, to trust that even their deepest secrets and darkest fears can become fertile soil for tender new seeds to flourish.[1]

For most of our three hundred thousand years on this earth, humans were intimately connected with her. Many researchers point to the 1950s as a marker for when that connection eroded, with the advent of television. Other researchers point to the scientific, political, and economic revolutions of the seventeenth and eighteenth centuries. Western culture's dualistic, hierarchical worldview has led to the belief that we are the most important beings on this planet. The ontological distinction between subject and object that has disconnected us from our natural environment has led to the damage we have done to the earth and all the beings that inhabit it. Regarding the earth and its many resources as an object that we are entitled to exploit for power and gain has wreaked irreparable damage, and it has also cut us off from a deeper, sensory connection with the earth and with ourselves.

The earth and all the beings that inhabit it will benefit from the subjective relationship of interconnection and interdependence. The earth is our teacher. We learn from the rhythms and cycles of change. We experience belonging, security, and stability. We develop a healthy sense of danger to guide our actions, and open up to earthly pleasures. We can spread our roots wide and reach deep into the earth. Walking in the footsteps of our ancestors, we feel our connection with the earth and the beings that share the earth with us. We pledge to live in harmony and be good stewards for future generations.

The following questions can guide you to experience the earth element subjectively.

1. If weather permits, go outside. If not, look out a window. As I look out my window, I ask my Parts that see things that need to be taken care of to relax, to give me space to experience the space around my home in a different way.

2. With the intention to appreciate and enjoy, use all of your senses for several minutes while you notice your inner bodymind responses. Your eyes may see the dirt, the plants, maybe a few animals. Your ears may notice sounds. Your nose may take in smells. If you are outside, you may feel tactile sensations. Walk on the earth without a destination.

3. What body sensations are you aware of?

_____

_____

_____

4. Are you aware of Parts? Does this connection with the earth connect you with your Embodied Self energy? How do you notice this?

_____

_____

_____

5. Name some of the gifts you have received from the earth.

_____

_____

_____

6. Consider all the other beings right now living on this earth. Consider all those who have lived on this earth before your birth. What sensations are you aware of?

_____

_____

_____

7. As, or if, you feel gratitude and a desire to give back, find a way to nonverbally express these feelings.

_____

_____

_____

8. In what ways do you give back to the earth?

_____

_____

_____

Because trauma burdens tend to cause our energy to rise upwards in a vortex, and may even numb the lower part of our bodies, Somatic Awareness—associated with the earth element—can help with grounding physically and metaphysically. Self energy is available to us in the world around us, not only from other beings but also the ground we stand on. The earth has nourished us and has been a solid place of belonging for millions of years. It even holds the bones of our ancestors. The following exercise assists with grounding, which is crucial to support our deeper explorations.

EXPERIENTIAL EXERCISE
GROUNDING AND BEING NOURISHED BY THE EARTH

1. You may want to practice this exercise in different positions—sitting, standing, or lying down. If you are lying on your back, bend your knees so your feet can press into the floor.

2. Bring your awareness to the places in your body that directly connect with the ground or the floor. Stay focused on these sensations for several moments, letting go of any unnecessary muscle tension.

3. Consciously invite your body to rest down. Connect with your gratitude for the gifts and support from the earth.

4. Imagine roots spreading from the places in your body that are touching the ground, extending in any direction. Through these roots, you can release burdens to the core of the earth where they can be absorbed by magma and recycled, or you can receive qualities from the Self energy in the earth to flow throughout your system.

5. You can extend this rooted experience by imagining you are a tree. You might want to stand, look at a tree, and mimic it. Imagine your roots extending deep and wide through the soil, taking in the water and nutrients through your trunk and drawing this nourishment upwards towards the highest twigs. You can bend with the wind and reach for the sun with this secure connection with the ground.

6. Does this exercise help you heighten your awareness of your Self energy? How do you notice it?

7. List a few of the gifts the earth has given you throughout your lifetime.

8. Research has shown us that gratitude is associated with a host of physical and mental benefits, such as improving sleep, mood, and immunity, and decreasing depression, anxiety, and chronic pain. As you stay with your gratitude towards the earth, what do you notice happens in your body?

9. As gratitude wells up, it naturally leads to reciprocity, a desire to give back to the earth. Invite the words, pledges, and commitments to be in harmony, respect, and stewardship of our planet and all the earth's beings.

Noticing and appreciating the earthy aspects of our bodies can repair much of the ways individual and societal traumas have hurt our bodies. We can recover the truth of our bodies, that regardless of any physical limitations or beliefs our Parts have about our bodies, they are quite resilient, powerful, and intelligent, exhibiting all the qualities of Self energy. Bringing awareness to the fleshy, solid, earthy aspects of our body (including the muscles, fascia, and bones) may be useful for feeling more grounded, strong, confident, and present.

EXPERIENTIAL EXERCISE
CONNECTING WITH OUR EARTHLY BODIES

1. Lying on the floor, take a few minutes for your body to rest down into the surface, noticing your sensations as you settle in.

2. Bring a focused attention to your bones. First, your long bones—the femur, the long bones of your thighs. The two long bones of your lower legs. The long bones of

your upper and lower arms. Feel the weight of gravity on them. Imagine the spongy layer of marrow at the core of your bones that are right now producing millions of blood cells.

3. Now bring your focus to your flat bones. These bones protect your internal organs—your brain, heart, pelvis. The skull has many flat bones. If you are lying on your back, the weight of your head is resting on the occipital bone. In your torso, you find the scapula on the back body and your sternum on your front body. In your pelvic area is your sacrum.

4. Bring your awareness to your small bones. Begin above your sacrum to focus for a moment on every individual vertebra until you get to the occipital bone. There are typically twenty-six vertebral bones in the adult body. There are also twenty-six bones in the hands and the feet. Bring your awareness to each of these tiny bones and how they connect with each other through the joints.

5. Flesh is attached to all these bones. Take a moment to connect with and appreciate all your strong, hardworking muscles. Invite them to move how they want to move to be noticed and appreciated. Then let them rest and lengthen.

6. Come to a sitting, standing, or hands-and-knees posture that will allow for movement to feel your bones and muscles more fully.

7. Woven throughout your bones and muscles is your fascia. Fascia is a thin band of fibrous connective tissue that wraps around and embraces every bone, muscle, organ, nerve fiber, and blood vessel in your body. It shapes the body like an elastic sheath. The collagen in your fascia provides strength, stability, and flexibility. When stressed, it tightens up, restricting movement and causing pain. Fascia connects all the body systems, enabling communication and collaboration.

8. To bring awareness to your fascial network, begin to try out some gentle stretching movements. Listen to your fascia to get a sense of which movements feel good and right. You may find some places that feel knotted up, stuck, sore, or stiff. Take a pause. There may be a story to be heard. There may be a gentle movement this place would appreciate. Does tuning into your fascia connect you with your body as a whole?

Our Three Sources of Grounding

As discussed, life experiences can interfere with our ability to be grounded with the earth, leading to disconnection, instability, and insecurity about belonging. By revisiting the sequential path of our experience connecting with the earth—through the navel, pelvic floor, and feet—while being aware of sensations that arise, we can find those interferences and restore this ability, securing a reconnection with the earth.

The first place of grounding, of connecting with a source of nourishment, is our navel. Shortly after conception, the embryo grows a stalk from the front body that attaches to the uterine wall. All the resources for life flow back and forth through this umbilicus. Months after birth, the typical path of motor development leads to the infant sitting upright. This stable, balanced relationship with gravity allows for upper body developmental movements. In time, the infant pulls their body upright to stand and balance on their feet.

The following exercise brings awareness to these three places of grounding to find sensations that may indicate Parts that were interrupted in their motor development, restoring the full capacity to stay grounded or easily return to a grounded state when life events threaten to unseat you or pull the rug out from underneath you.

You may want to stop after each step to record sensations that may indicate a burdened Part as well as pleasurable sensations. You may want to stay with one of the three areas of grounding to explore Parts that missed out on a safe and secure grounding experience. As you bring your compassion to those Parts, together you can discover how to provide the experience that was missing for those Parts.

EXPERIENTIAL EXERCISE
REVISITING INFANT GROUNDING

1. Find a comfortable way to lie on the floor on your stomach. Take the time you need for your body and mind to surrender to the surface below as fully as possible. Scan for any muscles that feel they need to hold you up. Let the weight of gravity pull your bones and all the attached muscles towards the floor. Notice and name any sensations, or lack of sensation, that arise.

2. Imagine being enveloped in a warm ocean, attached through your navel to a welcoming, safe, and loving presence, connecting either to the womb, the earth's center, or both. Just as in the womb, nourishment can be received, and what is no longer needed can flow outwards where it will be taken care of. What sensations are you aware of? What were you able to let go of?

3. Let these sensations guide your movements. You might want to extend and flex your body, twist and turn, roll from side to side, from front body to back body. Eventually, find a way to come to sitting.

4. Sit either cross-legged on the floor, or move to a chair that allows your spine to be directly over your pelvis and your knees over your feet. Focus on all the places in your body that make contact with the surface below, especially the sitz bones of your pelvis. Bring awareness to the pelvic bones of the sacrum and tailbone as well as the muscles of the floor of your pelvis. Do your spine and head feel the support from below?

5. Play with your balance as your pelvis is rooted to the surface, to discover where your body feels best supported by gravity. Imagine your roots reaching from your pelvic floor

deep into the earth, receiving all you long for, drawing it upwards through your body, and letting go of what is no longer needed.

6. Note any sensations or Parts. Also, what did you receive? What did you let go of? What has changed?

7. Come to standing with your knees soft. Wiggle your toes, rock front and back, left and right, lift and lower your heels several times. Push down with your big toe, little toe, and heel. Scanning upwards from your feet, make any subtle changes in your alignment that will support this balanced connection with the earth. Experiment with taking a step in any direction, pushing down with one foot, and then the next.

8. Notice and name any sensations, or lack of sensation, that arose during these steps. Do the sensations point to Parts that may have experienced some challenges to a safe, secure connection through your navel, pelvis, or feet and legs?

9. Reflect on what these exercises showed you about your system's relationship with receiving nourishment, connection, support, stability, and belonging. Were you able to help any burdened Parts find a new, satisfying experience of connecting with the earth?

Restoring and Fostering Our Somatic Awareness

From the exercise above, you see that sometimes the body sensations inform us about a Part. It might be that the Part can only be found and known through the body. Moreover, the Part's entire story might be told as we stay with the sensations with an open curiosity.

Other times, our sensations are not the nonverbal communication of a Part, but rather our bodies letting us know what needs to be attended to. In either case, the practice of Somatic Awareness can help us restore the Self-led embodiment that is our birthright.

Deep within us, under the layers of hurt, lies a yearning to be freed from the shroud that covers the aliveness inherent in every cell and body system. As we develop our *subjective knowing* of our body, without judgment or analysis, we can let go of the wounds from the *objectification* of our body.

The next exercise will continue to explore how our awareness *of our bodies* can enhance our awareness *in our bodies*.

EXPERIENTIAL EXERCISE
AWARENESS *OF* ENHANCES AWARENESS *IN*

1. Get into a comfortable position that will support your full attention for about fifteen minutes.

2. Again, scan your body. Choose one place in your body to bring your focus on.

3. Why did you choose this part of your body?

4. As you were guided to explore your hand in the "Objective and Subjective Awareness of the Body" exercise at the beginning of this chapter, bring your awareness as fully as possible to this part of your body. Notice how you are feeling towards this part of your body, and ask any efforting Parts, concerned or judging Parts, distracting or analyzing Parts what they might need to take a rest and make space for your open, mindful attention to this place.

5. Notice anything that comes to you, such as sensations of the skin, muscles, bones, circulation, energy flow, temperature, weight, and impulses to move. Name the sensations.

6. You may want to draw a body map to illustrate your sensations. You can include the color and shape of your sensations.

7. Shift from being aware of these sensations to centering your attention within these sensations.

8. When you feel complete, notice if there are any changes to this part of your body from these several minutes of focused attention. Name the sensations. Would you say that these sensations indicate that this part of your body feels more alive, more awake, more aware?

Clinical Application of Somatic Awareness
Somatic Awareness with a Client

Awareness itself is transformative. The client's sensory abilities are awakened. Their relationship with their body begins to shift. The vulnerable Parts whose stories are locked in the body can emerge. The implicit memories and the preverbal attachment trauma are communicated through the body. The therapist not only hears the story but can read the body story being told through posture and facial expressions. The Parts' verbal story and body story become one coherent narrative and are fully witnessed by therapist and client. The burdens are released, and the client can more fully inhabit their body. Awareness of their body leads to increased awareness in their body, in every cell and system of the body. Somatic Awareness leads to restoring and cultivating Embodied Self energy.[2]

Somatic IFS therapists' goal is to bring a state of Embodied Self energy to their clients. Somatic Awareness helps us know when our internal system is led by Parts or by our Self. We bring Self to our Parts so they can trust Us to be in the therapist chair.

You have discovered that being grounded and in a harmonious relationship with gravity supports the flow of Embodied Self energy. You intentionally make a few changes in your posture, inviting the earth's energies to flow upwards from your feet and your seat.

If some slight tension or postural alignment lets you know that a Part is present, even a well-meaning therapist manager Part, you can give an appreciative nod to the Part. The Part senses your energy and begins to relax and trust You. You feel open to the relational field of energy and information flowing between you and your client.

The Self energy flowing through your body is communicated and transmitted nonverbally. It is reflected in your posture, facial expression, tone, and the pacing of your voice. You feel open to creativity and collaboration. Your client's state is also communicated and transmitted nonverbally. You stay calm and curious during some of the more challenging aspects of therapy, like when the client's Parts seem stubbornly blended in their system, and when you and your client both feel stuck and unsure of what to do. Being with your client in this relational field with Embodied Self energy, your pace slows down to "body time."

Somatic Awareness involves our perception, including *interoception* (awareness of our internal system) and *exteroception* (awareness of the external world). The Somatic IFS therapist uses interoception for awareness of their internal system, and invites, responds to, or directs the client's internal awareness of their bodymind system. What is perceived is then interpreted for meaning.

Parts and the Self perceive and interpret their perceptions differently. For example, a Part's exteroception perceives the therapist's facial expression as scowling, interprets this through their burdened filters as the therapist is a threat, and has an internal reaction of a racing heart and rapid breath. This autonomic nervous system response fuels a behavior in the client, like avoiding, defending, or attacking, which is likely to activate a Part of the therapist. The therapist uses their interoception to notice the activation in their system, and as their Parts separate, they bring curiosity and compassion to their client's behavior to unpack the cycle of perception-interpretation-activation.

The somatic exercises in this chapter hone our interoceptive abilities, noticing the ever-changing shifts in our sensations and energy throughout our bodies and how they are the source of many of our own as well as our clients' thoughts and emotions.

The practice of Somatic Awareness also develops our exteroceptive abilities as we focus as much, if not more, on our client's nonverbal communication. We are also aware of our client's exteroception. Remember, communication is about 90 percent nonverbal. While listening to the client's speech, we track *how* they speak as well as *what* they speak, just as our clients are tracking our nonverbal messages. Most of the communication between therapist and client is unconsciously received and recorded subcortically, where it affects us but is not available to inform our interventions. With the intention to listen to the whole story, we bring awareness to the client's nonverbal language and support their Self-led interoceptive awareness.

When in relationship, our awareness tends to shift externally, overriding our interoception. Losing a bit of ourselves is a common relational habit, as a Part imagines the person we are with will not feel us present with them if we are also aware of what is happening in our own bodyminds. The opposite is true. When we are more present with ourselves in each moment in relationship, we are, well, more *present.* Another habit is to focus primarily on our client's verbal stories—*what* they say more than *how* they say it.

Focusing on working somatically with clients shifts the habitual way we relate to our clients. Participants in my trainings practice listening to the verbal story of the client, the nonverbal story of the client, and their own inner states—each taking one-third of their attention.

EXPERIENTIAL EXERCISE
PRACTICING NEW LISTENING HABITS

1. Choose a program to watch on TV that you imagine will engage you emotionally. Mute the audio, turn off captions, and focus on the characters' postures, facial expressions, gestures, and any other nonverbal language. Another option is to watch a program in a language you don't understand so you can also hear the tone and pace of the voices.

2. List the body sensations you notice in your body as you watch this program.

3. Name the emotions you imagine the characters are feeling.

4. What specific bodily behaviors do you observe that indicate this? What Parts do you sense they are speaking and acting from?

5. Choose another program and practice listening to your own body sensations and the nonverbal communication of the characters simultaneously. You might find your awareness oscillating between the two ways of listening, or find one way of listening more challenging than the other way.

6. Practice this way of listening with a willing friend. Let your friend know you will ask them to share something important with you for about ten minutes. During this listening, you will be focusing primarily on your body and what you notice about their nonverbal language as they speak. Take notes on what you notice.

7. What body sensations are you aware of?

8. What do you notice about your friend's gestures, facial expressions, posture, movements?

9. Share this list with your friend. Invite your friend to share their experience of being listened to by you in this way, and ask if they are interested in knowing what you noticed in your body and what you noticed about their nonverbal expression.

10. You and your friend might want to switch roles.

Beginning a Session with Somatic Awareness

The Somatic IFS therapist can utilize Somatic Awareness to help with the beginning steps of a session. When the client responds to a question with sensation words, stay with the client's words that describe their physical sensations: painful, tight, tense, tingly, itchy, heavy, numb, empty, tender, weak, jumpy, and so on. If the client uses language that does not describe a physical sensation, ask them to stay with that word and see what sensations describe it. You can also suggest other words and inquire if they fit. Follow your Self-led curiosity as well as the client's.

GETTING STARTED WITH SOMATIC IFS

Below are some examples of how the therapist can use Somatic Awareness with a beginning session:

1. To turn the client's attention inwards, "What do you notice happening in your body . . . as you sit here with me? . . . as you tell me what is concerning you?"

2. For contracting, "Is there something you feel in your body that tells you it would be OK to work with this today?" "Is there any response you notice in your body that may mean there is some doubt or concern?"

3. To find a Part, "As you stay with this sensation, does it seem to be coming from a Part that wants our attention?"

4. To focus on the Part, "Where is the sensation?" "What is the depth, the size?" "What are the edges of this sensation like?" "Is there a pull with this tension?" "What is the direction of the pull?" "Is the energy sluggish or moving?" "What is the movement of the energy?" These questions serve to focus on the sensation, and the answers may not be relevant.

5. To flesh out the Part, "Are there thoughts/words/emotions/images that go with this sensation?" Or, if the Part shows up first as thoughts/words/emotions/images, the therapist can ask, "Are there any body sensations you are aware of that come up as you talk about this?" "Would it be OK to listen to what your body might be telling you about this?"

6. To befriend the Part, "How are you feeling towards this sensation/Part?" "Where in your body do you feel this quality?" If the answer reveals a sufficient presence of Self, "Maybe this openness/warmth/presence can flow to this Part in your body."

7. For connecting Part to Self, "As You send your Self energy to this Part, what happens?" "How does this Part respond?" "What happens in your body?"

Staying with the sensation can be challenging to the system. Occasionally check with the client to see if this is getting to be too much, and track for signs of the client moving towards being overwhelmed or shutting down.

When a Client's Parts Block or Restrict Somatic Awareness

Clients may let us know verbally that they can't or won't follow our suggestions to notice their bodies. They might compliantly agree, but there may be nonverbal signs: agitated body movements, increased tension anywhere in the body, a fast pace in their speech, a blank facial expression, shallow or rapid breathing, difficulty in hearing or understanding, behavior that is distracted, sleepy, unfocused, narrating, analyzing, or agitated.

1. Are there other behaviors you have noticed from clients that indicate a protector Part?

   _____

   _____

   _____

2. Recall a session when you sensed your client had difficulty bringing awareness to their body. Did any Parts come up for you?

_____

_____

_____

3. If so, explore the Part or Parts—sensations, beliefs, behaviors, feelings? What does the Part need from you to relax and trust you?

_____

_____

_____

The section in this chapter titled "When Our Parts Fear Somatic Awareness," helps us to bring a Self-led connection to these protector Parts. Although we understand their job is to protect us from pain, the price of suppressing our pain is suppressing our aliveness.

A client of SIFS staff member Beth Rogerson, whose Parts have used her body in extremely negative ways to get her attention throughout her life, describes her Part's fear of body sensations:

> My Dissociator Part has served me well for years! For years, I have *had* a body, never *been* a body. I have ignored signals that have resulted in important body functions ceasing to work. . . . Once I *do* sense into the body, it usually scares me. What *is* this sensation? It's since long forgotten and I need to get to know it. It's like a stranger living inside me. Is it a friend or foe? I have so far found that they're all friends. But when I meet them, I'm still not sure.

Helping Protectors Trust Somatic Awareness

Appreciate their efforts to protect. Respect them, and circumvent shaming Parts that may layer onto these protectors. We therapists humbly admit we don't know if the external or internal systems are ready to engage in this practice of Somatic Awareness. If the protectors are willing and open, we can offer exercises and experiments to find out more about these Parts and what they might need to find safety and to trust that the situation might be different today. We respect when the answer is "no" or "enough for now." Some of the following questions, either directed to the client or to their Part, may be helpful with fearful protectors. The Part's answers and responses may be verbal or nonverbal.

- "I understand you don't want me to pay that kind of attention to my body. I'm not going to try to force or trick you. I would like to get to know you better."

- "How are you feeling towards me as I say this?"

- "What do you believe could happen if I were to bring more awareness to my body?"

- "I agree that would not be a good thing to happen again to you."

- "What was that like when that did happen?"

- "Would there be any place or sensation in your body that would be OK to notice, maybe for just a short time?"

- "How would it be to just focus on the sensation and ask the emotions, memories, and thoughts to wait?"

- "What do your Parts need from you or me to trust it is safe to be aware of your sensations? How about if we take it very slowly, in small steps over time? If I watch carefully for any signs of this becoming too much for your Part?"

- Ask the Self of the client: "What can You tell the Part about what may be different now?"

- "Would this Part be willing to stay close by, to stop us if it needs to, and know we will check with it afterwards?"

Appreciate any "small" steps. Titrate. Acknowledge the courage and energy required to do this inner work. Suggest frequent pauses, breaks, and rests. These are a crucial part of the healing and integration process. Urgent, impatient Parts easily override the system's pace and rhythm and interfere with the healing process. Invite verbal sharing about what you have done so far, and what they might want in the future.

In time, as we appreciate, respect, and befriend the protector Parts, they grant permission to bring Self awareness to the body. They come to see that awareness is not only tolerable, but also beneficial, even transformational. As the protectors make space, the vulnerable Parts kept hidden and protected are free to come into our awareness. They have their body story to show and tell us. As their story is witnessed and unburdened, the protectors can finally relinquish their demanding jobs and find rest, play, and enjoyment.

When a Client's Parts Take Over

One common challenge that IFS therapists and practitioners encounter is when their clients have difficulty accessing their Self energy. Although we know cognitively that everyone has a Self that may be blocked, buried, or pushed aside by Parts, when our clients' Parts seem to be intractably running their lives, our Parts can despair at ever uncovering that elusive, ephemeral Self.

By definition, trauma has overwhelmed the system, causing the aspects of the traumatic wound to fragment and separate. Accessing this traumatized state in the internal system can unleash a pandora's box of extreme and volatile emotions and overwhelming sensory information. Exiles are desperate to be able to share their traumatic stories and can hijack the entire system in order not to be locked up again. Protector Parts are determined not to let them throw the entire system into a chaotic mess. They react by slamming on the brakes, leaving the body, and shutting down.

To avoid this Parts-led cycle of escalating dysregulation, the Somatic IFS therapist can direct the client to focus solely on the somatic sensation or symptom. A client of Trish Attia and a participant in a recent Step 1 Somatic IFS program describes how Somatic Awareness has helped him when he is taken over by an anxious Part:

> Focusing on my body, beneath my neck, takes me out of my head and moves me into a different neural pathway. I am no longer in the worry loop in my thoughts. I am not fighting the thoughts but simply moving my attention elsewhere.

Below are some suggestions and examples to help the client focus on the sensation to prevent their Parts from flooding the system:

- "Let's stay with this headache that just showed up as you began to share your story. We will leave any thoughts, even emotions, for later. Right now, where do you notice the pain? If the pain could show itself, what would it look like?"

- "I know the story is important, and I want to hear it. For now, would it be OK to just stay with this sensation? We can let the sensation get even bigger."

- "As you remember this event, I notice your mouth becoming very tight and tense. Would you be willing, for now, to bring your full attention to the muscles around your mouth? Notice the direction the tension is pulling in. Is there a Part tightening your mouth? Let's notice how it does that. What happens if it moves in the other direction?"

- "I understand a Part of you is concerned about this sudden shakiness in your left arm. Let's see if that Part would be OK with you staying with the shakiness, just watching where it is, feeling the different paces and intensities throughout your arm, and to notice how the shaking changes over the next minute or two. Let it know it can be as big or as small as it wants to be."

Have you had an experience where focusing on a sensation in the body helped a client's Parts not take over their entire system?

_____

_____

_____

Somatic Awareness with Exiles

A somatic approach to healing the wounds of trauma has been well researched and documented. Bessel van der Kolk in his work *The Body Keeps the Score* tells us that trauma is not the past event but is the residue left by the past event in the sensory experiences in our bodies. Somatic IFS brings the light of awareness to the sensory experiences to allow the Part to release the residue of the trauma.

The Somatic IFS therapist understands that, often, the client's trauma is held in their implicit memories. As discussed, traumatic events often occur before the ability to understand or speak language—in the womb, during the birthing process, or in the first few years of life when survival is dependent on caregivers. Traumatic experiences are stored in the cerebellum and the basal ganglia where they are largely nonconscious and can't be verbally articulated. Even when trauma occurs when the brain is mature enough to store the memories in the hippocampus, the amygdala, and the neocortex, where they would be available to be retrieved and consciously shared as explicit memories, trauma can alter the memory processes so that the traumatic memories are recorded as sensory and affective imprints. It is this sensory and affective imprint that we seek to update with the Somatic IFS approach to the trauma stored in the body.

With permission from the protectors, the body stories of our vulnerable Parts—our exiles—are available for witnessing and unburdening. Exiles have been isolated, locked in our bodymind systems, desperate to be found, heard, and freed. Traumatized exiles have most likely experienced the whiplash of emerging with their overwhelming feelings and behaviors, and then getting forced back into lockdown. Their desperation may cause them to take over, again activating the fearful protector Parts.

As the path is paved for the Parts holding the deepest pain of the trauma to finally show and tell their stories, we remember another assumption of the IFS Model—that our exiled Parts can regulate with the presence of Self energy (that of the therapist, the client, or both). We reassure them that we indeed want to know everything about them, what has hurt them, and what they need from us. We invite them to become more embodied so we can know them fully. As we meet them with Self energy, we help them to share their stories in a way that does not reenact the original wound.

We direct the exiles to share their story slowly, one piece of the puzzle at a time. We not only tell them that we can help them show and tell their stories safely, but also calmly and confidently reassure them that we want to help them safely share the whole story. We also promise we will not forget about or abandon them again.

Often the exile's story is told nonverbally as sensation and frozen movement impulses. It may be conveyed in the tone, pace, and pitch of their voice. Additionally, it might be revealed in visual, auditory, and olfactory memories. Each of these aspects of the fragmented story are noticed, named, received, and integrated so the complete story can eventually be told and witnessed by the Self of the therapist and the client. Only then can they let go of the load they have been carrying.

As they begin to share their story, either verbally or nonverbally, we can help them moderate the intensity of the physical sensations or the emotional expressions. We might speak directly to the Part (examples below):

- "I really want to know all you want me to know, and I understand how eager you are to be understood."

- "I know how many Parts have kept you from sharing your story, so it makes sense to me that you feel it is now or never, everything or nothing."

- "You may not realize that you have more than an 'on-off switch.' You also have a 'dimmer switch' so you can shed a gentle light on the story."

- "I will help you to tell your full story, one piece at a time, so you know it is heard, and so there is time to digest it. Are you OK if we take it a bit more slowly?"

- "You have shared a lot. Let's take a pause to notice how this is for you."

The client of Beth Rogerson who shared how her dissociating protector Part feared her body awareness, above, goes on to share how her thinking Part with the verbal stories steps back so she can hear the body story of her exile. Beth has shared that this client is truly embracing the question of what story her body wants her to know:

> My Thinking Part is a master in making up stories. These stories are just that—made up. The body doesn't make up stories; it gives me information on the now and on the now connected to the then—I can learn something about burdens stored in my body. I'm slowly but steadily (*fast* does not work) learning to understand what my body is trying to tell me, what the sensation means.

Integration of Somatic Awareness
How Somatic Awareness Cultivates Embodied Self Energy

Somatic Awareness is the foundational practice of Somatic IFS. As the logo shows, it supports all the other practices, which flow organically from the awareness of our bodies. It is a practice Somatic IFS therapists incorporate into their daily lives to enhance their own embodiment. It may be the only practice utilized during a session as the therapist listens to their own sensations and what they observe in their client's nonverbal communication, and as they invite the client to tune into their own embodied experience of Parts and Self.

Much of this chapter has focused on how awareness of our sensations can reveal Parts that are using the body to do their jobs, attempting to tell their long-held stories, or both. When their burdens, stored in the flesh and bones, are released, the original qualities of the Parts are freed. In other words, the inherent Self of each Part is restored. The core, essential Self of the individual is freed up as well, and the Parts recognize and trust this Self to listen to them and lead the entire system with compassion, confidence, and wisdom.

This process requires Self energy to relate to the Parts. These words from Trish Attia's client describe how when he notices a Part, he first establishes Self energy within his system to welcome the Part:

> In moments of squeezing and self-consciousness and worry, I am drawn to first going inside and trying to give over an energy of openness to my internal world. The focus isn't on where the immediate anxiety is in my body, but first on creating a more spacious and welcoming sense, giving over a feeling of openness, and conveying that there is room internally for me and all my Parts.

What about the times when we cannot find that openness in our internal world? Parts need Self to heal, but Self needs Parts to heal before Self is available. It can feel like when we can't find our glasses because we need our glasses to find them. Often the therapist's Self is the only Self energy available in the room, but eventually, the client's Self emerges and the process of healing flows exponentially.

How can Somatic Awareness help us as therapists to access that Self energy even when our Parts are still weighed down with heavy burdens?

_____

_____

_____

EXPERIENTIAL EXERCISE
EMBODYING SELF ENERGY

1. We notice the Parts believing they need to take over our system, and we ask them if they are willing to wait while we create a safe and welcoming space for them.

2. Find a Part that is willing to wait in the wings while you find, embody, and enhance your Self energy.

3. Self energy is ineffable, but in teaching IFS, we have found words that describe some of the qualities of Self energy that begin with the letter C—calm, connected, creative, courageous, confident, compassionate, curious, clear. These are all embodied states. You may already be feeling one or more of these qualities. Are there sensations that go with this quality? Notice how it is to bring this quality to the Part you asked to wait.

4. Self energy is evident in our bodies in many ways. Like Trish Attia's client, our bodies might feel spacious and open. We may feel warmth in our hearts. We may feel grounded, centered, light, solid, and relaxed. We may feel energy flowing in our central channel. How do you typically experience Self energy in your body?

5. Turn your attention to your own body. Do you find any of these qualities in your body right now? If so, focus your awareness on the sensations there. Invite them to expand, to take up more of your body. Invite it to expand beyond your skin, as big as it wants to be. Does the waiting Part sense this energy?

There are situations that feel all encompassing, for which we need some immediate and effective way to access Self energy. My go-to is to connect with the ground below me. I feel my feet on the floor, my butt on the chair. That seems to send a basic message to my Parts to stay in the present moment. On an exhale, I send the reactivity of my Parts as far into the earth as possible, and invite the energies from the earth to fill my body. This helps my system to be grounded and connected to a source larger than "me." With this stable connection, I can more easily bring curiosity and compassion to the activating situation.

Somatic IFS staff member Beth ONeil focuses on her back body when she is aware her body is being activated by her Parts. When her front body is full from empathically resonating with the pain of her clients, she shifts her awareness to her back body. She leans back into her chair, feeling the sensations of her back body where it touches the chair. Resting back into the support of her chair, Beth's calm, connected, and compassionate presence is restored.

How do you quickly access Self energy when your Parts are activated?

_____

_____

_____

Trish Attia's client from earlier eloquently describes his experience of uncovering his Embodied Self as follows:

> As I go into my body with an attitude of acceptance, I strive to convey allowance and acceptance to all my natural movements. I try to get curious about how I can make even more space for the flow of energy. Allowing my moment-to-moment intuition to guide me—letting me know where more spaciousness and openness is needed. . . . The more I connect with my disowned Parts and make space for them, the more solid and larger I begin to feel. This often leads to a larger sense of self-embrace and confidence. . . . I am experientially connected to me with a sense of acceptance and worth. . . . I can untuck my shirt. There is room for all of me.

EXPERIENTIAL EXERCISE
MAKING ROOM FOR ALL OF OUR PARTS AND SELVES

Enjoyment is the intention of this exercise. However, you may want to allow some spacious time for the exercise, as some Parts may find the amount of time to be challenging in some way. Bring compassion and respect to any Parts that need to take this exercise in smaller doses. You can decide to pause for a break whenever you choose.

1. Start by letting go of all you have learned about paying attention to your bodies from yoga, meditation, qigong, fitness classes, even Somatic IFS. Let go of the intention to find a Part. Let go of thinking there is a right and wrong way to do this exercise. Let go of the idea that some sensations are good and others are not. Let go of directing your body—let it lead you.

2. You will be giving your full attention to your body for no reason at all. Simply because you can. Because you are alive. Because it is a good way to spend your time. Because it is fun to be surprised.

3. Let your body lead you to settle into a comfortable position. Bring your attention entirely to your bodily self.

4. Give your attention free rein to flow from your whole body to a specific area, to another area, and so on.

5. Watch your attention over time shift from being the observer of your body to *being* the sensations and energy as you experience them moment by moment.

6. If visual images arise, notice and welcome them.

7. Let your body lead your completion and reflection on this exercise.

Integration

1. Which of the exercises were especially helpful for you to experience the practice of Somatic Awareness?

_____

_____

_____

2. Does connecting with the earth help you access your Self energy?

_____

_____

_____

3. Did you find that staying present with the sensation of the Part helped it not to blend or take over?

_____

_____

_____

4. Were there any exercises that you want to remember so you can do them regularly?

_____

_____

_____

5. Which body sensations led to a Part that you want to continue to get to know?

_____

_____

_____

6. If you use the IFS Model and have incorporated Somatic Awareness into your sessions with clients, what have you noticed? Have you found any obstacles?

_____

_____

_____

7. If you do not use the IFS Model, how has this practice been included in your modality?

_____

_____

_____

Notes

1 Susan McConnell, *Somatic Internal Family Systems Therapy*, 49–50.

2 Susan McConnell, *Somatic Internal Family Systems Therapy*, 87.

3

Conscious Breathing

Purpose of Conscious Breathing

THE FOUNDATIONAL PRACTICE of Somatic Awareness naturally leads to the second Somatic IFS practice, Conscious Breathing. Aware of our body sensations, we soon notice our breathing. We can bring a more intentional consciousness to the largely unconscious and generally involuntary behavior of breathing. Conscious Breathing reveals our current physiological and psychological states and helps us shift our internal systems towards more Self energy. Often, Self energy is just a breath away. This piece of a poem by Sufi mystic and poet Rumi describes the two ways breathing is considered in Somatic IFS:

> There is one way of breathing that is full of shame and constriction. Then there is
> another way: a breath of love that takes you all the way to infinity.

Traumatic burdens of "shame and constriction," as well as fear, sadness, despair, and rage lying in the dark corners of our psyches, may be revealed in our breathing patterns. Conscious Breathing breaches the divide between consciousness and unconsciousness, and addresses these burdens with the IFS Model. In this way, Conscious Breathing offers a path that takes us, if not all the way to infinity, in the direction towards more Embodied Self energy. Relying on the rooted connection with the earth and our capacity for body awareness, we breathe in the air and the energies from the space around and above us. We feel the flow of Self energy connecting us with the earth and sky through our central channel as we breathe "a breath of love" to our Parts and the wider world.

In the "Grounding and Being Nourished by the Earth" exercise in chapter 2, you may have imagined yourself as a tree, firmly rooted to the earth, able to bow to the wind as it makes the limbs dance and the trunk bend. You may have felt some qualities from the earth able to flow through your body. The practice of Conscious Breathing completes our relationship with above and below. The energies from above and below flow through our bodies from toes to head and from head to toes, through our central channel. Our posture becomes more aligned. The muscles that had been fighting the force of gravity relax. Self energy flows from the earth's core through our bodies and beyond.

Beginning to read this chapter, your breathing might not have been in the forefront of your awareness. Of the twenty thousand or so breaths we take in a day, we are not conscious of most of them. When I remember to bring consciousness to a few of my breaths, I feel more awake, clearer. If I am having trouble falling asleep, a few minutes of awareness of the sensations of my breathing may be all I need. When I am irritated, my breath can help me pause, and perhaps avoid a snarky reaction. Sometimes breathing reminds me that the world is much vaster than my Parts perceive and I can breathe out my concerns.

If you would like to take a pause in your reading, you can stand up and enjoy a few breaths to give your body, mind, and eyes a little break. Research has shown that simply bringing awareness to our breathing for even a few minutes has positive outcomes on our heart rate variability, blood pressure, and mood. With this next exercise, notice your bodymind states before and after.

EXPERIENTIAL EXERCISE
A LITTLE BREATHING BREAK

1. Standing, take a deep in-breath. On the exhale, draw your navel in towards your spine and up towards your heart.

2. Lift both arms as you breathe in, and return your arms to your side as you breathe out.

3. Gently twist your torso, allowing your arms and hands to freely move.

4. Lift and lengthen the front body on the inhale as the back body shortens. Fold and curl the front body on the exhale as the back body lengthens.

Individual Application of Conscious Breathing
Vertical Alignment

Our posture reflects and determines our inner bodymind system. Messages like "sit up straight" add to our pile of burdens of objectification. Our breathing supports and is supported by our dynamic inner alignment. Our inner alignment, in turn, supports our Self energy. Receiving Self energy from the earth, we open to Self energy from the sky. Our crown chakra, the place at the top of our heads that as infants was our soft spot, is considered a portal to welcome these energies from the sky, sun, moon, stars, planets, galaxies—to flow within us.

EXPERIENTIAL EXERCISE
RESTORING THE VERTICAL FLOW OF SELF ENERGY

1. Sitting or standing, recall some of the exercises from chapter 2 that helped you feel grounded. Allow your spine to lengthen, your tailbone and shoulder blades to drop. Feel the weight of gravity and find the alignment that supports your body with the least effort. Lift your body from your seat or feet through the crown of your head. Invite your body to let go of any unnecessary tension.

2. Imagine Self energy from the core of the earth flowing upwards through your body.

3. Consciously breathe in the air from the space around and above you, feeling the air as it travels in and out through your body. Imagine you are breathing in air from your crown chakra and out through your feet or seat.

4. Feel into the central channel in your body. It might be a beam of light, or a flow of energy through your torso. Take a moment to sense and visualize this channel and notice how your bodymind organizes around it.

5. What is the size of this channel?

6. Do you feel energy flowing through this channel?

7. What is the direction?

8. What is the force of the flow?

9. Are there any restrictions in the flow?

10. Take some moments for awareness, reflection, appreciation.

11. Are there any changes in your body? In your emotions? In your breathing?

Structures of the Respiratory System

- Muscles:
  - The diaphragm is the major muscular player, providing 80 percent of the inhalation force. This large dome-shaped muscle attaches to bones at the front, back, and sides. On the inhale, it takes a plate shape as it contracts downwards. On the exhale, the diaphragm relaxes, returning to its dome shape.
  - The thoracic and abdominal muscles expand on the inhale, relax on the exhale.
  - The intercostal muscles and muscles of the face, mouth, pharynx, neck, and upper chest are also involved in the act of breathing. The pelvic diaphragm expands and condenses with the breath.

- Nervous system:
  - Structures in the brain stem, the pons and the medulla oblongata, control our unconscious, involuntary breathing. They detect a buildup of carbon dioxide, sending messages to our respiratory muscles via spinal circuits that cause the diaphragm to relax, restoring normal pressure in the chest cavity, and forcing air out of the lungs.
  - The autonomic nervous system (ANS) and cortical structures of the brain are engaged when we bring conscious awareness to our breathing.
- Organs and pathways:
  - Nasal cavity and sinuses, soft palate of mouth, lungs, alveoli, bronchial tubes, trachea, larynx, pleural membrane, blood vessels.
  - Our soft palate and pelvic diaphragm expand and condense with the breath.

EXPERIENTIAL EXERCISE
EXPLORING THE ANATOMY OF RESPIRATION

1. Breathe naturally for several breaths, following the path of the air.

2. For the next ten breaths, follow the sensation of the inhale—drawing air into the nostrils, the nasal cavity, passing down through the throat via the trachea, larynx, bronchial tubes, and upper, middle, and lower lungs.

3. For the next ten breaths, follow the sensations of the exhale as the air reverses its path—the lower, middle, and upper lungs, bronchial tubes, larynx, trachea, nasal cavity, and nostrils.

4. Bring your hands to explore the movement of bones as you breathe in and out—the sternum, collar bones, spine, and ribs on your front, sides, and back.

5. Bring your hands to explore the movement of muscles as you breathe in and out—the diaphragm, intercostals, abdominal muscles, and neck—your front, sides, and back. Notice any unnecessary muscle activation—around the eyes, jaw, and muscles of your pelvic floor—and ask these muscles to relax.

Air Element

We become aware that the air surrounding us is the same as the air inside us, and that the Self energy inside us is the same as the Self energy around us. This mutual synergistic exchange of both gas and energy is the universal dance of our essential unity and interdependence.[1]

My internal system often needs to be reminded that Self energy does not exist just in my system. When I have difficulty accessing it, and other Self-led beings are not around, my breathing can remind me of the Self energy all around me. The air element reminds us, as does the earth element, of our interconnection and interdependence with all living beings. We depend on the precious oxygen for our survival and appreciate plants, especially the vast rainforests, as we enjoy the reciprocal relationships between animals and plants. Our reliance on oxygen bonds us with every other animal. We pledge to protect our air, knowing that our actions will affect living beings for many generations.

Our air brings us far more than oxygen. Wind, rain, snow, thunder and lightning, the sun, moon, stars, planets, and the vast infinite reaches of the cosmos offer many qualities long associated with this element. Intuition, imagination, inspiration, liberation, lightness, openness, and clarity are a few of the qualities. Moreover, air is associated with the heart chakra. The air, just as the earth, is a Field of Self energy that we can open to as it surrounds, informs, and nourishes us. We breathe in from this Field, receiving guidance and inspiration, and we breathe out, releasing what we no longer need. We can also send our Self energy into the world on our out-breath.

Attention to our breathing makes us more aware of the air that surrounds us. The vastness of this space appears to our senses to be empty, but physicists tell us that empty space is not really empty, that the seeming void is seething with energy and particles that flit in and out of existence. Also, regardless of our sensory experience, we learn that physical phenomena, at the subatomic level, is nearly entirely empty space. We associate "empty" with nothingness. The emptiness referred to is considered the ultimate healing force, linking all beings in a network of energy exchange.

With the first Somatic IFS practice, we experienced the solidity of our bodies. With this second practice, we experience the immense emptiness of our bodies. We experience it subjectively as spaciousness. When our Parts inhabit places in our bodies, we feel dense, tight, heavy. A few breaths sent to those Parts, the "breath of love," can restore spaciousness and lightness to our bodies.

EXPERIENTIAL EXERCISE
THE AIR ELEMENT

1. You may want to go outside for this exercise, but inside is also fine.

2. Using all your senses, what do you notice about the air?

3. What body sensations are you aware of?

4. What emotions are you aware of?

5. Does your breathing change?

6. Grounding into the earth, take some deep, slow breaths. Are there any shifts in your inner system as you intentionally breathe in the air?

7. Bring awareness to the infinite space that surrounds you—front, back, sides, and above. Reach up with your arms, stretching your sides, lengthening your back. Let your arms and head reach, stretch, and move in all directions.

8. Bring your awareness to your central channel. Open your crown chakra. Invite the positive, healing energies of the air to enter you through your nose and then through the top of your head. As you open to receiving qualities from this air element, what qualities do you notice?

9. Do you associate those qualities with Self energy?

10. Can you invite the qualities you are experiencing to expand, to be amplified?

11. As you breathe in and out, consider all the beings who are right now breathing in and out too.

12. Consider all those beings who have breathed their last breath.

13. Opening to the air and the infinite space beyond may welcome wisdom from guides and ancestors. Are there any images, thoughts, words, movement, or sensations that come to you from this element?

SAFETY GUIDELINES

As you do the exercises in this chapter, if you begin to feel overwhelmed, activated, or dissociated, take a pause to bring your attention to the safety in the present moment. Come back to the exercise when you feel grounded, curious, and calm. You may choose to do the exercises with a partner or a therapist.

Finding Parts—Protector Parts, Vulnerable (Exile) Parts
FINDING PARTS IN HABITUAL BREATHING PATTERNS

When I remember to focus my attention on my breathing, the longer I stay with my breath, the more I realize how my habitual breathing practices cheat me of the fullest aliveness available to me. I begin to breathe more into my back body. My in-breath becomes slower and deeper. Maybe it is the increase in oxygen, but I feel calmer and clearer. My awareness goes to places in my body that are hurting, weak, or stiff. My in-breath naturally flows to those places. My exhale allows me to settle in and rest. I feel the Parts that have served me all day to keep functioning slough off my body. Some days, I feel relaxed. Other days, I feel the heaviness in my heart, actually in my entire torso, that had been masked by my busy, functioning Parts. If I stay with Conscious Breathing long enough, the heaviness melts.

We may find that intentionally taking a few breaths can help us shift our attention from our external situation towards our internal systems. As we breathe in the air around us, we feel more spaciousness in our bodies and inner systems. Connecting with the Self energy from above and below, we explore our habitual breathing patterns to find, focus on, and befriend Parts. Concentrated Conscious Breathing may gently invite these Parts into the open space our breath brings to our inner systems. Every hour, we take almost one thousand breaths, most of which we are unaware of. Yet our Parts are behind the scenes, affecting our breathing to fulfill their protective roles or tell their stories. We can bring consciousness to these Parts through Conscious Breathing.

EXPERIENTIAL EXERCISE
CONSCIOUS BREATHING TO ACCESS YOUR INTERNAL SYSTEM

1. Take a few breaths without intentionally changing your breathing. You may notice that your breathing pattern tends to change simply from your awareness, but do your best to observe your natural breathing pattern with open curiosity. Ask any Parts that distract you or have judgments or concerns about what they need to trust you.

2. Follow the sensations as the air enters your nostrils and travels up into your nasal passages, then down through your trachea and into your lungs. Follow the sensations as the air leaves your lungs, reversing its direction to finally leave your nostrils and enter the air.

3. Does attention to these few breaths help you shift your awareness from your external to your internal world?

4. How do the sensations of the in-breath differ from the out-breath?

5. Where in your body do you feel movement as you breathe in and out?

6. Is your breath more in the upper or lower part of your torso?

7. Is your breath more in the front body, side body, or back body?

8. Describe the depth and pace of your breathing.

9. Do you notice any restrictions in your breathing? Where?

10. Stay with one aspect of your habitual breathing that you are curious about, again without trying to change it. As you focus on it, be open to thoughts, feelings, images, or sensations elsewhere in your body that may be connected with this breathing pattern.

11. Take a few more breaths, noting any changes in your breathing, body, thoughts, and feelings.

12. Do you notice Parts, Self, or both?

13. Experiment with some breathing patterns to find which ones help you more fully feel your Self energy. Is this breathing different from your usual breathing?

PROTECTOR PARTS AND CONSCIOUS BREATHING

Our breathing patterns are constantly affected by our emotional states, making our breathing patterns a valuable way to identify our Parts. These Parts may have been, like our breath, lying outside our conscious awareness. Our protector Parts affect our breathing so we won't become overwhelmed or shamed by our strong emotions. They have found that restricting our breathing works well to keep us from crying, screaming, fighting, and feeling the pain from neglect, abuse, loss, and betrayal. The protectors tighten our diaphragm, intercostal muscles, and abdominal muscles to control our air intake and restrict the exhale so our breath is shallow. They tighten our jaw and pelvic floor and affect our posture, all of which in turn affects our breathing. Many of these behaviors are an inherent, adaptive response to trauma from our ANS.

Before you focus on your typical breathing patterns to see if you find a protector Part affecting your breathing, first notice what happens to your breath when you intentionally tighten your jaw. What happens when you tighten your pelvic floor muscles? When you round your shoulders, slouch your front body? What happens to your mood as your breathing changes?

EXPERIENTIAL EXERCISE
FINDING PROTECTOR PARTS THAT CONTROL OUR BREATHING

1. Bring to mind a recent situation where you felt sad, afraid, or angry, and it did not feel safe to express this feeling. Invite the Part that did not want this feeling to be expressed to show itself to you in your body energies, posture, facial expression, and sensations. Give it some time to fully embody.

2. What happens with your breathing?

3. Let this Part know that you understand that it uses your breathing to do its job, containing your emotions.

4. Ask your protector Part if it wants you to understand more about how, when, and why it felt it had to contain your emotions through your breath. What is it afraid would happen today if it did not do this?

5. What does this Part need from you to let go of the restriction?

6. As you relate to your protector Part, have the restrictions on your breath been released?

7. As an experiment, you can also ask the muscles involved in respiration to relax, to allow your breathing to be fuller and deeper. What happens to this emotion?

VULNERABLE PARTS (EXILES) AND CONSCIOUS BREATHING

Our breathing patterns may point us to the vulnerable Parts that are carrying the brunt of the wounding for the internal system. Rapid breathing may indicate a fearful Part, while shallow breathing may lead to a depressed Part. Noting differences between the in-breath and out-breath may even reveal Parts with birth trauma. As with their protectors, the ANS is the source of the exiles' breathing patterns. Our earliest traumas are recorded subcortically, affecting the muscles and neurons central to our respiratory behaviors. Bringing consciousness to our habitual breathing patterns can reveal their presence and histories.

Their story may begin at birth as they took their first breath of air. If born prematurely, the infant may have experienced some respiratory distress. Oxygen deprivation during birth may leave a lasting imprint on the breathing pattern. Infants and toddlers may reflexively hold their breath from fear, pain, and shock, even to the point of losing consciousness. Vestiges of this reflexive behavior can be locked up in the nervous system and in the respiratory muscles and organs currently involved in our breathing.

The breathing patterns in infants develop sequentially as their central nervous system matures. Once the diaphragm's position is established, this muscle synchronizes with the pelvic floor, strengthening the baby's core to eventually stand and walk. Any disruptions during this developmental process affect the nervous and respiratory systems.

Bringing awareness to restrictions on our in-breath may tell the story of a Part with a belief about not being deserving of receiving. A Part that wants to die will not want to open to the fullness of the inhale. Another Part may carry the belief that the outside world is dangerous or toxic. "Taking in" might also be infused with a sense of danger.

Restrictions on our out-breath might tell the story of a Part having to hold in and not let go. A full out-breath can feel like a harbinger of death. Anxious, insecure Parts can be expressed in truncated exhales, leading to hyperventilation. Depressed Parts may be found in shallow breathing. Trauma can result in what is known as paradoxical breathing, where the actions of breathing are reversed. The diaphragm moves upwards during inspiration and downwards during expiration.

As an experiment, you can purposely adopt one of the following Parts-led breathing patterns to find the emotions and beliefs associated with the pattern.

SAFETY GUIDELINES

Note your bodymind responses to each of the breathing patterns. These breathing patterns can elicit powerful emotions, so try them for a few breaths to get the information you want, and then take some deep, slow breaths to help your system return to calm.

EXPERIENTIAL EXERCISE
INTENTIONALLY TAKING ON A PARTS-LED BREATHING PATTERN

1. Restrict your inhale with shallow breath, rapid breath, breathing mainly with your upper lungs.

2. Restrict your exhale—shallow, rapid, shorter than the inhale.

3. Shallow, rapid breaths with both your inhale and exhale.

4. Paradoxical breathing—on the inhale, draw your navel towards your heart. Breathe into your upper chest. On the exhale, push downwards with your diaphragm. Do this for only two or three breaths.

During our lifetimes, we have experienced pain and shame that was too much to process at the time. These burdens are stored in our bodymind systems, including our respiratory systems. Traditional Chinese medicine associates the lungs with loss and grief. We all have experienced loss in our individual lives as well as globally. Since my book was published in the spring of 2020, over seven million people have died from COVID-19. Many more have died from other diseases, accidents, armed conflicts, and other forms of violence. We are witnessing and experiencing violence against people of color, Jews, Muslims, LGBTQ+ people, and other marginalized groups. Blocking the expression of our sadness affects the smooth action of the lungs to receive and let go and to send Qi (Self) to the rest of the body. It is important to release the protectors from their roles and allow the Parts waiting in our lungs to safely express the immense grief stored there. IFS has taught us that exiles can share their stories, with some coaching, in a titrated way so that the protectors won't feel a need to distract or otherwise interrupt the process.

Before having the intention to find one of your vulnerable Parts in your breathing patterns, access your Self energy. There may be Parts activated by the paragraphs above. You may find Parts that want to find something, or Parts that fear finding something.

SAFETY GUIDELINES

Connect with the energies from above and below, as establishing your vertical alignment will be very helpful. Also consider doing this exercise with a friend or a therapist.

Remember, your Parts can let you know from your breathing if you need to take a break. Rapid, shallow breathing will tell you your nervous system is activated and your Parts need to be comforted by You.

EXPERIENTIAL EXERCISE
OUR VULNERABLE PARTS AND BREATHING PATTERNS

1. Focus on your inhale and exhale. Notice the rhythm, pace, depth, and location of your breath. How is it to take in air and to let it go? Notice the moments between the inhale and the exhale.

2. Stay with anything about your observed respiration that most interests you.

3. As you stay with this, do you feel any emotions?

4. Are there thoughts, images, memories, or other body sensations?

5. If a Part emerges, send your Self energy to the Part—through your words, breath, or touch. Let the Part know how glad you are it has shown itself to you.

6. What else does this Part want you to know?

7. What does this Part need from you?

Conscious Breathing Includes Specific Breathing Techniques

The exercises above focus on Parts-led breathing habits and how applying the IFS Model to these Parts can free them from these patterns. The practice of Conscious Breathing also includes specific breathing practices to cultivate our Self energy and bring greater well-being to our bodymind systems.

Many of these breathing practices can be used specifically to help notice, regulate, and shape the state of our ANS. The vagus nerve oversees our respiration. Often a change in our breath, of the pace and depth of our breath, signals to us that a Part has been triggered by an external event or an internal message. We perceive we are in danger and our ANS shifts into fight, flight, freeze, or fawn, affecting our breathing in different ways. When the pace of our breath tells us our ANS is in sympathetic activation, we can use the practices that slow our breath, prolong our exhalation, and restore full, calm, balanced breathing. When we are in the parasympathetic dorsal vagal state, feeling sluggish and spacey, our breathing rate slows and gets shallower. We might find the Bellows Breath, or gently sipping several times on each in-breath, restores our energy.

Consciously and voluntarily making shifts in our breathing can help us access Self energy. The slow, deep rhythms of a few breaths bring a soothing presence to our internal system. We can connect our heart energy with our breath because our hearts are nestled intimately between the lungs. The rhythms of the heart and our breathing gently rock the Parts. Our Self energy can flow on our breath to the places in our body where we find our Parts.

There are some techniques that are like first aid for when our burdened Parts are dominating the airwaves. A change in our breathing tells us a Part has taken over. We can make a choice to direct our breath in a different way. We can inhale, pause, exhale, and pause. We can take a long inhale and an even longer exhale. A pause at the end of the exhale allows the lungs to release a bit more air, making room for a deeper inhale. It helps to count the breath, such as counting to four for the inhale, the pause, and the exhale, or a longer count for the exhale and the pause before the inhale. Breathing in through the nose and out through pursed lips is also helpful for regulating the ANS.

There are also breathing practices that can foster more Self energy over time and bring many health benefits to our bodies. Yoga has introduced many of us to powerful breathing techniques with their pranayama practices, with many benefits for our mental, physical, and spiritual well-being. I have shared several of these in my therapy and teaching, and I include them here: Nadi Shodhana (Alternate Nostril Breathing), Bhastrika (Bellows Breath), Bhramari (Humming Bee), and Ujjayi (Ocean Breath), among others.

You can start with a few minutes of practice each day. As your bodymind system adjusts, you can increase the duration and frequency. You will discover that some of the exercises help you relax, some are soothing, and some are enlivening. All the exercises begin with you sitting in a comfortable seated posture with a straight spine, shoulders relaxed. You can choose how many rounds of each exercise feel right to you at this time. As you complete an exercise, let your breath return to normal.

SAFETY GUIDELINES

Note any changes in your internal bodymind system in the space provided at the end of each exercise.

EXPERIENTIAL EXERCISE
ALTERNATE NOSTRIL BREATHING

1. Bring your right hand up to your nose.

2. Close your right nostril with your right thumb and inhale through your left nostril.

3. Pause, then close your left nostril with your ring finger and exhale through your right nostril.

4. Inhale through your right nostril, pause, then close your right nostril and exhale through your left nostril.

_____

_____

_____

EXPERIENTIAL EXERCISE
BELLOWS BREATH

1. Inhale through your nose. Exhale forcefully through your nose as you draw in your abdominal muscles.

2. Inhale forcefully through your nose and expand your abdomen.

3. Exhale forcefully again, contracting your abdominal muscles.

4. Continue this cycle with an equal emphasis on inhale and exhale.

_____

_____

_____

EXPERIENTIAL EXERCISE
HUMMING BEE

1. Close your eyes. Close your ears with your thumbs and gently place your index fingers just above your eyebrows.

2. Inhale deeply through your nose.

3. Exhale slowly while making a humming sound like a bee.

4. Focus on the sound and vibration created by the humming.

_____

_____

_____

EXPERIENTIAL EXERCISE
OCEAN BREATH

1. Inhale deeply through your nose, expanding your belly and constricting the back of your throat. Pause at the top of the inhale.

2. Exhale through your nose, drawing your navel towards your spine and constricting the back of your throat.

3. Close your mouth and inhale deeply through your nose, pause, and then constrict the back of your throat to create a hissing or ocean sound (like Darth Vader).

_____

_____

_____

EXPERIENTIAL EXERCISE
THREE REGIONS BREATHING

1. Place one hand on your mid-chest and one on your abdomen just below your sternum.

2. Inhale your breath all the way to your abdomen. Feel the air press against your hand. Exhale from your abdomen and feel your hand rest down.

3. Breathe your air first into your belly, feeling it lift your hand on your abdomen, then feeling it lift your hand on your mid-chest, and finally feeling your air filling your upper chest.

4. Exhale first the air from your upper chest, then your mid-chest, and finally your abdomen.

_____

_____

_____

EXPERIENTIAL EXERCISE
DIRECTING YOUR BREATHING IN YOUR LUNGS

Direct your breath in your lungs: Breathe in and out three times for each, followed by a return to your natural breath for three breaths.

- Direct your breath to the right lung, then the left lung.

- Direct your breath to your back body, then your left and right side body, then your front body.

- Direct your breath to your upper right lung, then your middle right lung, then your lower right lung.

- Direct your breath to your upper left lung, then your middle left lung, then your lower left lung.

_____

_____

_____

Embodied Speech with a Partner

"Speech" in Somatic IFS is not limited to the verbal content. Generally speaking, our speech is obviously verbal communication, but how we speak—the timbre, tone, intonation, volume, rhythm, pitch, pace, and resonance of our voice—conveys far more than the content. Our speech is dependent on the same anatomical structures as our breathing. Speech involves the diaphragm, lungs, trachea, larynx, nasal passages, sinuses, and the muscles controlling the soft palate, tongue, and lips. We speak on the exhalation as the air is expelled and goes over the vocal cords in the larynx, which close together and vibrate. The sound of the voice depends on the tension and length of the vocal cords. Our posture affects our respiration and, therefore, our speech. If burdened Parts are determining our breathing, they also certainly affect our voice quality.

Collective vocal sounds of humming, singing, and chanting have been used for centuries as a way to express and release emotions. Some of our Parts' stories can't be told in words, but freeing the voice to be expressed in creative ways can restore voice to the silenced, exiled Parts. Sounds naturally accompany our expression of emotions. We sigh, scream, moan, growl, yell, laugh, and groan, unless our Parts inhibit them. The sounds themselves stimulate the vagus nerve and bring health in many ways to the bodymind system. They create more coherency. The sounds touch the minute colloidal particles suspended in the fluids of your body—blood, lymph, and the extracellular matrix (ECM).

This next exercise can be done with a partner, or with a therapist, to restore your embodied speech. You may find other creative ways to free and express sounds.

EXPERIENTIAL EXERCISE
HUMMING WITH A PARTNER

1. Begin by lying on your back on the floor. Let your body feel completely supported by the floor. Feel your body relax.

2. Bring your awareness to your breath. On your exhale, tighten your vocal chords slightly. You will hear a slight sigh as you breathe out.

3. Relax your jaw, and with your lips gently touching, hum on the exhale. Where do you feel the vibration?

4. Hum, feel the vibration, rest, then hum some more.

5. Send your hum to places in your body that are not vibrating.

6. Play with different volumes, pitches, and rhythms. Pause frequently to notice changes in your body, and what sounds your system likes best.

7. Slightly open your lips to experiment with additional sounds, comparing each one. Soft vowels of *aahh, oohh, eehh.* Long vowels of *aay, eey, iiyy, ooh.*

8. Add a consonant to the beginning of these vowels, such as *V, M, P, N, K, T, R, L, S.*

9. Add a consonant to the end of the vowels, such as *M, N, L.*

10. Find someone close to your own size and sit back-to-back.

11. Take turns humming. One hums, the other feels the vibration and then hums in response. Play with different sounds.

12. Hum together as in a duet, each noticing their own and their partner's vibration and sound. Take some pauses.

13. For completion, each can make sounds that express this experience.

14. Share your experience verbally with your partner, using Embodied Speech.

Clinical Application of Conscious Breathing
Using Conscious Breathing with a Client

As therapists, we begin with awareness of our own systems, our interoception. We have discovered that bringing consciousness to our breath before and during the session both reveals Parts and helps us return to more Self energy. We typically find manager Parts that need to know, try to get it right, and worry they won't be good enough. These Parts may tighten and brace the muscles of respiration, causing the breath to be shallow and contained. Our breathing may suddenly increase during an intensely emotional session.

Staff member Lesley Hartman shares how she uses this practice to get back in touch with her Self when she is in the therapist role and her Parts get activated:

> The most effective thing for me is to send my presence to my Parts on my breath. The experience of this for my Parts is like being surrounded by spaciousness and welcomed. They feel surrounded by a womb of Self presence in the air around them. It's like a felt sense of: "I'm all around you; it's OK for you to be here too." My Parts receive the message much more quickly than if I internally tried verbalizing those things, which I used to do prior to practicing Somatic IFS.

Another thing I find helpful is to focus on the crown of my head. For some reason, I always feel some element of my connection to Universal Self energy; to Self as wave, through the crown of my head. I then allow that sensation of connection to flow down to wherever the Parts are in my body.

EXPERIENTIAL EXERCISE
THERAPIST RESTORES THEIR SELF ENERGY

1. Imagine you are sitting in your office with a client that you find challenging. Invite a memory of a particular situation that activated your Parts.

2. Stay with this memory, recalling all the details and finding the Parts that were activated.

3. Do you notice any changes in your breathing?

4. Check your posture and make any shifts to establish your inner vertical alignment.

5. Inhale deeply, and then exhale slowly and completely for several breaths.

6. Direct your in-breath to where you find your Parts in your body. Breathe out your Parts' activation.

7. Bring your awareness back to the situation with the client that you found challenging. How are you feeling towards this client now?

8. With your Self energy restored, how might you address this challenging situation?

Using Conscious Breathing in a Session

Coordinating our breath with our client's helps us get a sense from the inside of what our client is experiencing. We breathe in their inner state and resonate with it, and we send compassion on our out-breath. Simply inviting our client to bring awareness to their breath can be transformative. In addition there are many breathing techniques that can facilitate every step of the IFS process.[2]

SETTLING IN/GOING INSIDE

Because the breath is a bridge between inside and outside, between what is conscious and what is unconscious, we may suggest a client take a breath or two and let that breath take their attention inwards. Examples:

- "To help go inside, you can start with simply noticing your breathing. Just follow the sensations and movement as you breathe in and out a few times."

- "Let your in-breath draw your attention inside; on your out-breath, you can let go of whatever was taking your attention before."

- "Let's prepare this space to be for you and the work you want to do today. As we feel the floor supporting us from below, we breathe out and draw our navel towards our spine. With each out-breath, your shoulder blades and sacrum can drop down and your spine can lengthen. Notice how your ribs expand as you breathe in—your front, sides, and back. Enjoy the rhythm of your in-breath and out-breath. Breathe in spaciousness, and let go of anything you no longer need as you breathe out. This space you have created is for you. We can open to guidance from this space below and above us to help our work today."

FINDING A PART

Remember, Somatic IFS therapists use exteroception, such as observing our client's breathing, and invite the client's interoception. The client's breathing may reveal a Part that becomes the focus of the session. Connecting with the client, we notice this—the rhythm and pace of their breathing, how it moves the body. We continue to use our exteroceptive abilities to find Parts as we track our client's breathing patterns throughout the session and invite the client's awareness. When working virtually, it is important to be able to see some of the client's torso as well as their head and neck. Clients, in turn, learn to track their breathing as a way to find their Parts in session and in their daily lives.

Some therapists fear that acknowledging these body-based behaviors may be shaming to our clients. Culturally, we may have learned it is impolite to bring attention to our naturally occurring bodily behaviors. If this does occur with a client, we can help them work with that Part that feels shamed. This rarely happens, though, when acknowledging behaviors is delivered heartfully. Usually our clients appreciate knowing that we are paying such good attention to them.

- "I am noticing your breath is fast and shallow. Are you aware of it too? Stay with that."

- "You tell me you can't take a deep breath. Let's bring our curiosity to this. Let your in-breath gently touch the place where your breath feels restricted. Do you sense a Part that is needing to keep your breath shallow?"

- "I understand that your shallow breathing has helped you find a Part of you that is feeling anxious. Keep breathing into the place of restriction to let this Part know we are aware of it."

- "I noticed you stopped breathing right after you said that. Could that be letting us know another Part of you does not want us to be with the anxious Part?"

- "This Part has told us it wants to get rid of your anxious Part. I notice you are breathing faster as you share this. Let's try taking a deep breath, and a longer exhale. Pause after the exhale for a second, then take another slow, deep in-breath. So now we know there is an anxious Part, and another Part that wants to get rid of it. How are you feeling towards each of these Parts?"

- "Let your breath tell both Parts you are glad you have found them, and you will listen to each of them."

FOCUSING ON AND FLESHING OUT THE PART

Directing an in-breath to the place in the body where the client has located their Part can help the client keep their focus on the Part. Our breath brings spaciousness to allow the Part to show itself more fully—the thoughts, images, emotions, and memories as well as other Parts it relates to.

- "Let your breath gently touch the place where you feel the tension in your belly to let this Part know you are here with it."

- "As you breathe your Self energy to that Part, what happens with the tension? Keep breathing into your belly. Let your breath tell the Part you will stay with it. Breathe out any distracting thoughts."

- "As this Part feels your spacious attention, what happens in your belly?"

- "Let this Part in your belly know you welcome anything it wants to show you or tell you about itself—words, thoughts, a picture, or a memory."

FACILITATING A RELATIONSHIP WITH THE PART

When the client is feeling Self energy towards the Part, they can breathe that energy towards the Part, surrounding and embracing the Part with the client's compassion, clarity, and confidence.

- "Bring your awareness to your heart, which is nestled between your lungs. Take a deep, full breath into your heart. Send your heart energy to this Part on your exhale."

- "Breathe your Self energy to this Part as you inhale. Are there words that go along with the breath that your Part needs to hear?"

- "Let's see what happens when you bring your breath to this Part in your body. How does this Part respond?"

- "What happens with your Part as it knows I am breathing along with it?"

CONSCIOUS BREATHING WITH BLENDED PARTS

When clients' Parts believe they need to take over, as is a regular occurrence, it can frustrate both the client and therapist. Narrating protectors may dominate, or anxious, agitated Parts may flood the system. Shifting the client's focus to their breathing begins the unblending process. Awareness of the breath, and counting the breaths, lessens the anxiety.

Until the client's Parts unblend, the therapist can be the source of Self energy. The therapist can briefly synchronize their breath with that of their client for a few breaths and note how that impacts their internal system, giving them information about the client's internal system. Returning to a balanced, full breathing, the therapist can breathe in the energies of the client's Part and send compassion on the out-breath. The therapist can suggest one of the breathing practices described in this chapter. Directing the client to breathe as they would in a Self-led state regulates the nervous system towards a ventral vagal state, lowers blood pressure and metabolism, and increases mental clarity.

- "What do you notice about your breath right now? Would you be willing to try a different way of breathing to see what happens with this Part that is taking over?"

- "It seems your breath is mostly in your upper chest. Can you stay with that, and then experiment with gently bringing your breath into your lower lungs? What is happening?"

- "Take a full breath. Pause. Take an even fuller, longer exhale. Pause. Let's do that for three more breaths. How are you feeling now?"

- "I will time you for a minute while you count your breaths. Can we try one more minute? Your breathing has slowed down. How is that anxious Part right now?"

- "I would like to hear the rest of the story, but I'm noticing your breath is becoming faster as you speak. Do you notice that? What is your breathing saying to you about how you are feeling right now?"

BREATHING TECHNIQUES FOR SHIFTING THE ANS STATE OF THE CLIENT

- More rapid, shallow breaths indicate sympathetic activation. Slower breathing, longer exhalations, diaphragmatic breathing, and purse-lip breathing can shift this ANS state to ventral vagal.

- Slower, shallow, irregular breathing indicates a dorsal vagal parasympathetic state. Shift the ANS to sympathetic or ventral vagal state with resistance breathing, a deep breath followed by a sharp inhalation or exhalation, and yogic Breath of Fire.

- Support automatic yawning and sighing.

BREATHING TO SUPPORT SHIFTS IN THE SYSTEM

During the course of a session (or sessions), as Parts are found, known, and helped, there are many moments of "aha"—of satisfaction, relief, surprise, even joy. We track the breath throughout sessions for changes in breathing that indicate these moments. We notice a deep, easy, slow breath, sometimes accompanied by a sound, a sigh, or laughter. We acknowledge and highlight these spontaneous bodily responses to support the transformations.

- "I see you just took a deep breath. That looks like it feels good. Let's take another one together."

- "Did you notice how your breath slowed down when your Part felt your presence?"

- "As your Part feels relieved, I hear a sigh coming on your out-breath. Can you let that out?"

- "Aah, good. I see a big yawn. Stay with that. How do you feel now?"

DRAWING UPON THE AIR ELEMENT FOR UNBURDENING

Conscious Breathing can restore Self energy to the system, making space to allow the Parts' stories to unfold and be witnessed. The burdens can be released to dissolve into the infinite space through the exhale, and through various sounds and embodied speech. The unburdened Parts can breathe in all the gifts of this air element to reinstate the original roles and qualities of the protectors and the ones they have protected.

- "Breathe air—or the energy from the infinite space above you—into this dark, cramped, stuck place in your body. Do you feel more spaciousness there now?"

- "Can that darkness ride out on your exhale? Are your Parts OK with letting go of all of what has been stuck there? Can the air take the darkness to the farthest reaches where it can be dissipated?"

- "Breathing into this new space, what qualities can float in on your breath?"

CONSCIOUS BREATHING WITH THE INTEGRATION STAGE OF SOMATIC IFS

We celebrate the transformation of habitual breathing patterns. We breathe in gratitude to Parts that dared to trust. We check for Parts that have concerns about the change. Specific breathing practices may be suggested for follow-up.

- "How is your breathing now? What else changes in your body now that your breath is full, slow, balanced?"

- "Can you breathe in that gratitude and appreciation you just spoke about and send it to your Parts?"

- "Would you like me to send you the breathing technique that helped you today so you can practice it this week?"

EMBODIED SPEECH WITH CLIENTS

The therapist's voice is crucial in conveying a calm, safe presence to the client. A slower pace invites the space that nonverbal Parts require—"body time."

> Nothing reveals our Parts like the tone of our voice. We may not be aware of our tone when we speak. We can track our clients to gauge whether the tone, pitch, volume, and rhythm of our speech is inviting the ventral vagal state of social engagement or perhaps is activating the ANS arousal of their Parts.[3]

Remember, Somatic IFS considers the importance of Embodied Speech with the therapist's communication to convey Self energy. The "Humming with a Partner" exercise in the "Individual Application" section above can help foster Embodied Speech, and the therapist can also record a session to assess the quality of their speaking voice.

Listening to the quality of the client's speech gives us information about their inner world. Changes in pace, rhythm, pitch, volume, and tone may reveal a Part. For example, when a client responds to our question of "How are you feeling towards this Part?" with curiosity or compassion, the therapist may assume the Self is talking, but something in the client's voice may hint that it may be a Part.

Below are examples of how a therapist may use voice to help a client separate from Parts and communicate from Self. These interventions, when the therapist is in Embodied Self, can be empowering, even fun, rather than a correction or criticism.

- "Your words are powerful, yet as I hear you say them, it sounds to me like a Part is speaking rather than You. Can you hear that too?"

- "As I hear you say that, it sounds to me like it may be a Part that is saying that rather than You. Can you hear that too?"

- "Where do you feel the compassion in your body? Breathe into that place and let the word come from there."

- "What do you notice in your body as you say 'No!'?"

- "Now that your Part that has been gripping your diaphragm and tensing your throat feels my presence, is it willing to experiment with saying 'No'?"

- "Let your diaphragm relax, allowing for a deep inhale. Breathe into that place in your body where you find the 'No!' that wants to be spoken. Let's start with another sound and work up to the 'No.' On your exhale, tighten your vocal cords and let out a sound. I can do it with you if you would like."

- "Let's experiment with different sounds (hums, sighs, growls, various vowels, pitches, tones, volume, length). *Aaahhh, ooooh, eeeeh, uuuuhhh.* Now let's try a consonant in front of your favorite vowel sound."

- "Which one of these sounds feels right? How can you tell? Do you want to say 'No!' or is there a different sound, word, or words? Are your other Parts OK with you voicing this?"

Integration of Conscious Breathing

We have experienced how bringing awareness to our breathing patterns reveals Parts, and that simply shining the light of awareness on these Parts can make a shift in both our breathing and our Parts. With Parts no longer needing to use our breathing to do their jobs or tell their stories, our natural breathing patterns are restored, bringing healing to the entire bodymind system. We make new neural connections and restore the subcortical motor control patterns in the central nervous system. We have more mental clarity and concentration, greater endurance and resilience, and improved digestion and immunity.

1. Was there a particular aspect of your breathing that interested you?

_____

_____

_____

2. What did you discover about your habitual breathing patterns? Did it lead you to find a Part? If so, what did you learn about your Part? Is it a protector or one of the vulnerable ones being protected?

_____

_____

_____

3. Is establishing your inner vertical alignment helpful for your breathing? For embodying Self energy?

_____

_____

_____

4. Was there a breathing technique you found especially helpful to shift your ANS? To foster Embodied Self energy? Is it a technique you want to practice in the future?

_____

_____

_____

5. Did you find any exercises helpful for restoring your Self energy when a Part takes over?

_____

_____

_____

6. If you are a therapist, what did you find most valuable about using Conscious Breathing in your clinical practice?

_____

_____

_____

Having experienced the first two practices of Somatic IFS, Somatic Awareness and Conscious Breathing, we are rooted in the solid earthiness of our bodies and opened to the spaciousness of our inner system. Our inner vertical alignment allows the energies from above and below to flow throughout our system, providing an anchor as we step into the relational field.

We breathe in, and our bodies expand. We breathe out, and our bodies condense. Not only do we feel calmed by the rhythm, but we also receive life-giving oxygen on the in-breath and release what we no longer need on the out-breath. Oxygen and prana nourish the heart nestled between our lungs. Aware of the vast space around us, we are open to receiving guidance from this seeming void.

Breath is a bridge in many ways. Breath bridges the conscious and unconscious, the material and nonmaterial, the interpersonal and intrapersonal. It connects our bodymind and Spirit and Soul. It unites our inner and outer worlds and connects us with all living beings who depend on the same fragile air. Our breathing is a universal dance of our essential oneness. It returns us to the present moment, again and again, the only place we can find Self. This bridge of Conscious Breathing takes us to the next chapter, where we explore the rich, complex relational realms with Radical Resonance.

Notes

1 Susan McConnell, *Somatic Internal Family Systems Therapy*, 98.

2 Susan McConnell, *Somatic Internal Family Systems Therapy*, 121.

3 Susan McConnell, *Somatic Internal Family Systems Therapy*, 108.

4

Radical Resonance

Purpose of Radical Resonance

THIS CHAPTER FOCUSES on relationships at every level of system. Radical Resonance assists relationships among the Parts of the individual's internal system (the intrapersonal); relationships between two people, in particular the therapeutic relationship (the interpersonal); and relationships among the collective (intergenerational, ancestral, and community).

The previous chapters bring the somatic practices of awareness and breathing to the intrapersonal system. We have come to know burdened Parts whose strategies and stories are embedded in our tissues and evident in our breathing patterns. We have met Parts whose role is to protect vulnerable Parts or protect the system from the shame and pain leaking out, and other protectors who try to get rid of or overpower other Parts. We all have a lot of Parts, as it turns out, and these Parts have developed a complex system of interrelationships. They polarize, protect, criticize, caretake, control, and compete for dominance. Some of them carry burdens; others are free of these distorted beliefs and behaviors and are connected and collaborative with the rest of the system. As our Parts come to trust the presence of Embodied Self, they are restored to their original nature, and inner harmony is restored. At least intrapersonally.

As we enter the realm of *interpersonal* relationships, where two inner systems interact with each other in ways similar to our internal systems, things get more complex. Often, it is my interpersonal relationships that reveal my burdened Parts. I may easily congratulate myself for being so Self-led (finally), until I am confronted with someone who I (my Parts) perceive to be annoying, critical, controlling, accusatory, or threatening. My humility restored, I remember to connect with the earth for stability and belonging, and the air for spaciousness and insight. I breathe in Self energy to my Parts. In time, I am ready to move back into the horizontal field of relationships and attempt to repair the rupture.

This practice of Radical Resonance is truly radical, as it gets to the root of trauma and attachment wounds from conception to the present. It can repair and reshape the neural firing patterns in the brain and revise other chemical and energetic patterns in the body. Resonant relationships harness neural plasticity and our inherited hardwired impulse to make somatic shifts in relation to another person.

Individual Application of Radical Resonance
Our Resonant Bodies

Our entire bodies are resonant. Every sense organ, cell, system of the body, various fluids—all are receiving information and energy from the outside world. Much of this information is communicated nonverbally, from one right brain to another, involving the ANS, amygdala, insula, mirror neurons, bonding hormones, social-emotional bias of the right hemisphere, and prefrontal cortex.

We are impacted by inanimate objects and living beings just as we impact others. The impact is measurable as vibrational frequencies. Before we enter the world of person-to-person relationships, you may want to experience your resonant body with an object. Ask any Parts with a desire to do it right, or a fear that they won't, to know there is no right way. You probably will not feel the "vibrational frequencies" mentioned above. Let your senses be open to a new experience, freed of their usual ways of seeing, listening, smelling, touching, and enjoy the experience.

EXPERIENTIAL EXERCISE
RESONATING WITH AN INANIMATE OBJECT

1. How do each of the actions below affect you? Which of your senses bring you the most resonance?

- Seeing: Cover your eyes with your hands to relax them, then open your eyes to gaze at a picture on your wall, or out the window. Let the image come to your eyes rather than your eyes going towards the image.

- Listening: Notice any sounds in your environment. Try to avoid naming the source of the sounds. Listen to them as if you were at a concert. Let the sound come to your ears.

- Smelling: Take in the odor or fragrance of an object. Letting go of naming or evaluating the smell, allow it to enter your nasal passages, possibly your mouth. Imagine the smell traveling from your olfactory nerve to your limbic brain. Are there any emotions or memories that come to you?

- Touching: Find an object near you to touch. Approach it as you would a newborn kitten. Close your eyes. Notice the temperature, texture, weight, and anything else that interests you about this object.

2. Which of the following physical sensations did you experience?

- ❑ Relaxation of your facial muscles
- ❑ Tingling or tremors that travel along the surfaces of the body
- ❑ Sensation in the eyes of tearfulness
- ❑ Warmth and openness in the heart
- ❑ Greater sensitivity in seeing, hearing, smelling, touching
- ❑ Movements, micromovements, rhythms, pulsations, vibrations

3. Was any part of this exercise activating for a Part of you?

4. Did you feel bored, get distracted, feel unsafe, or get overstimulated? If so, can you resonate with the Part and see what it needs from you?

5. If you did this exercise indoors, you may want to go outside and repeat these four activities.

Water Element

The water element is associated with this practice of Radical Resonance. This element is connected with the unconscious and the qualities of the right brain that assist our resonant capacity—intuition, emotion, empathy, and psychic energy. Water connects us. All living beings depend on it for life. And it teaches us about flow and connection.

Our bodies, like the earth, are largely made up of water. Most of the fluids in our bodies are in interstitial fluids, the extracellular matrix that bathes every cell. We speak of using our blood, sweat, and tears to achieve a difficult task. We also have lymph, cerebrospinal fluids, gastric juices, urine, semen, vaginal fluids, saliva, and mucus. These fluids are connected. They all have their own pulsations, their own rhythms. Connecting with the fluids in our bodies amplifies our resonant capacity.

Water dissolves barriers, sweeps away debris, cleanses, softens, purifies, and transforms. Water patiently and persistently wears away stone, drop by drop. Parts' burdens can dissolve as the Part feels resonance from Embodied Self. Just as the water in rivers, lakes, and oceans has the power to reshape the land, resonant relationships reshape the neural firing patterns in our brain and revise other chemical and energetic patterns in our body.

In whatever way a Part shows up in the body, Embodied Self can thaw out Parts frozen in our tissues, slake the thirst of Parts parched from neglect, restore the flow, and release emotions that have stagnated in the fluids of our bodies. With Embodied Self energy, we do not fear drowning in a trauma vortex. We fluidly and buoyantly absorb the frequencies of the Parts' pain and transmit the frequencies of Self energy to the Part with right brain-to-right brain communication. Fluids can become blocked by burdened Parts. Tuning in to the various liquids flowing through our bodies can increase our resonant capacity.

EXPERIENTIAL EXERCISE
EXPLORING THE FLUID NATURE OF YOUR BODY

1. Find a comfortable position. We have already experienced the solidity of our bodies with the earth element, and the spaciousness of our bodies with the air element. Considering that the human body is roughly an average of 60 percent water, give yourself the time you need to attune to your inner fluids.

2. Notice the following movements, rhythms, and pulsations of the fluids in your body. What are the qualities of each fluid?

- Cell: Lying down, get into a position that can help you imagine you are a single cell floating in a sea. Imagine your body is spherical and filled with water. Your skin is the membrane. This membrane is taking in what it needs from the water and keeping out what it does not want. It is giving to the water what it needs to let go of, and holding on to what it received from the water that it can use. You feel the expanding and condensing in your cell body as your wise membrane provides what you need for nourishment and protection.

- Blood: Feel the rhythm of your blood being circulated through your body—the arterial and venous flow, similar to the ocean waves. Take a few breaths to appreciate how your blood is loading and unloading oxygen and nutrients to every cell.

- Gastric juices: Bring your hands to rest on your abdomen. Tune in to the juiciness of your organs. You might feel subtle sensations of the peristalsis from your esophagus to your anus. Take a moment to appreciate how your gastric juices help with digestion and fight infection.

- Cerebrospinal fluid: Lying on your back, bring your hands to rest on your head. You may be able to feel a subtle movement in the bones of your cranium caused by the production and absorption of the fluid in your brain and spinal column. This rhythm is typically a bit slower than the breath.

- Lymph: Come to standing with soft knees to experience the flow of lymph, since it depends on muscle movement. Begin to gently bounce up and down from your knees, shaking your hands and arms from lower to higher.

3. While standing, tune into the fluid aspect of your entire body. Let your body move you to express its fluidity. Imagine you are a sea creature, with your internal fluids moving in a fluid world.

Radical Resonance and Our Body

The frequency of Self energy is transmitted, and the frequency of burdened Parts is transmitted. Especially in relational interactions, body-based attachment experiences are sent and received by way of our bodies. Much of this information may be outside of our awareness. It may be blocked or ignored by protector Parts. Regardless, it is impacting our relationships.

Every one of us, including those of us who carry the scars of early abuse or neglect, have within us Self energy. When we bring our Self energy to these Parts, our Self resonates with the vibrational frequencies of their pain and transmits Embodied Self energy to the Parts. We receive the early nonverbal stories. We witness and resonate with the vibrations of the sensations and emotions. The frequencies of Self energy can bring the burdened Parts' frequencies into coherence. The Somatic IFS practices free our own Embodied Self energy to be the secure attachment figure our young Parts have been yearning for. Self needs to be embodied to resonate with the frequencies of the right brain stories of our burdened Parts in order to rewire our habitual relational patterns.

Major Organs of Resonance: Right Brain, Heart, and Gut

- Right brain and limbic brain—mirror neurons and other limbic structures send information to the neurons of interoception, and allow us to sense from the inside out what the other person is feeling. Limbic structures attribute an emotional meaning to our body sensations.

- The heart is the strongest organ of resonance, producing magnetic and electrical impulses in the body five thousand times more powerful than the electromagnetic field created by the brain.

- The gut is regulated by the enteric nervous system, often called the body's "second brain." The enteric nervous system, a sophisticated neural network from our esophagus to our anus, is made up of some five hundred million neurons, thirty types of neurotransmitters, 90 percent of the body's serotonin, and trillions of bacteria (the gut microbiome) that are involved in bidirectional communication with the brain, linking emotional and cognitive centers of the brain. Commonly, we refer to "gut feelings," "gut wisdom," and "butterflies in our stomach" that suggest an intuitive knowledge flowing between this second brain and the first brain.

EXPERIENTIAL EXERCISE
GETTING TO KNOW OUR RESONANT BODY

1. Give an example of how your attuned attention to another person's nonverbal behavior gave you information about their inner world that the person did not verbally report.

2. What in your body told you this?

3. Focus on a person or being that opens your heart. Stay with the images, memories, feelings. What sensations do you feel in or around your heart?

4. When have you had a gut feeling about something that later turned out to be true?

5. Do you have a Part that is reluctant to trust your gut knowledge?

EXPERIENTIAL EXERCISE
STEPPING INTO THE HORIZONTAL REALM OF RELATING

1. Start by connecting with earth and sky: Standing, bring your focus to the sensations in your feet. Bring your attention upwards from your feet to your legs, pelvis, spine, torso, and head. Send your roots downwards and do any movement that helps you feel more grounded and anchored. Feel into the space around you. Breathe this in through your nose and the top of your head. Imagine, or feel, the energies from above and below flowing through your body. Which qualities of Self energy are you feeling?

2. Horizontal Field: Imagine there is a person in front of you that you have a relation-ship with. You might choose a compatible, loving relationship, or a more challenging one. Close your eyes and see that person in front of you. How do you sense their presence?

3. Take one step forward towards that person. What sensations do you notice?

4. Does this lead to finding a Part? If so, what does this Part want you to know?

5. If you are curious to explore whether your system responds differently to different relationships, you can continue slowly and mindfully walking towards these imag-ined people. What sensations are the same, which are different? Are there different Parts with these different relationships? If so, what do they want you to know?

6. Return to where you were standing when you found your connection with the earth and sky. Feel the sensations you experienced. Let those energies flow through your system. Bring this Self energy from within and without to your Parts that showed themselves to you.

7. Which Parts were familiar? Which Parts were a surprise? Stay with each one of them until you can sense or hear what they might need from you.

SAFETY GUIDELINES

Track your body and breath to gauge your level of activation. Use any tools you learned in the last two chapters to return safety and calm to your inner system.

EXPERIENTIAL EXERCISE
RESONATING WITH A PART

1. Choose one of the Parts you met in the exercise above as you moved into the relational field that you will be able to hold in your compassion.

2. Invite the Part to become more embodied. Let it express itself in facial expressions, gestures, movement, sounds, and emotions. Give the Part as much time as it needs to let you know how it is feeling.

3. Thank the Part for showing itself to you through your body.

4. What did you feel in your body as you witnessed this Part?

5. Let this Part know that you felt it—seeing, hearing, moving, touching. Be specific. Communicate verbally and nonverbally with this Part. What happens with the Part as it hears, sees, and senses you?

6. Invite the Part to once again take over your body to show you how it is feeling now. How is it different? How is it the same?

Blocks to Resonance in the Body

We are hardwired for openness, to be impacted by others. But sometimes it can be too much. Resonating emotionally, physically, energetically, and spiritually is intimate and often risky. If we are not sufficiently resourced by our own or others' Embodied Self energy, then our systems can be overwhelmed by terror and grief.

Our protector Parts can erect a barrier that gives them a safe distance from others' emotions, causing us to feel numb, disconnected, dissociated, avoidant, distracted, or apathetic to another's pain. These reactions are also in our hardwiring. We typically have Parts that blame and shame us for the behaviors of our protectors. However, we can feel compassion for these Parts as we understand the source of their behaviors is in our vulnerable, open, sensitive Parts nearly drowning in overwhelming emotions. These burdens can be healed, and our resonance can be restored.

The burdens from blocked resonance are found in our bodies. Bodily fluids attract the energetic charge of the emotional overwhelm, becoming blocked or distorted, and these fluids are everywhere in our bodies, affecting every physical system. The burdens may also be found in or near the heart, with sensations of heaviness, numbness, and muscular tension. Intense grief, fear, and anger could result in the heart being stunned by adrenaline and other stress hormones, weakening the heart, leading to a condition called Takotsubo cardiomyopathy, or broken heart syndrome, which mimics a heart attack. The complex communication between our gut and our right brain is driven by the ANS. The reciprocal interaction of the gut-brain axis involves neural, endocrine, and immune functions. Overwhelming emotions can impact both our emotional ability to resonate and our digestive systems.

EXPERIENTIAL EXERCISE
PARTS WITH BLOCKS TO RESONANCE

1. Do You identify any of the above blocks in your body? Do You find a Part?

2. What are the Parts' behaviors? Do they use your body to block your resonance? Are any of the behaviors familiar to you?

3. Send your Self energy to one of these Parts. How does this Part feel towards You? Give it the time it needs to get to know You.

4. Can the Part show or tell You about the situation or environment that caused it to believe your natural resonance was dangerous or not welcome?

5. What does this Part need from You to let go of blocking your resonance?

Radical Resonance with a Partner

SAFETY GUIDELINES

Each partner is encouraged to consider their own self-care with the following partner exercises.

EXPERIENTIAL EXERCISE
RESONATING WITH A PERSON

Your partner will read the instructions below, and you will remain silent. You may want to have paper near you to record your responses. Your partner will read the instructions for the Individual Field, and then sit across from you to read the instructions for the Relational Field. For these partner exercises, you and your partner may want to each do the exercise, switching roles, and then share your experiences verbally and nonverbally.

1. Individual Field:

- Establish your inner vertical alignment, connecting with above and below, lengthening your spine from tailbone to head.

- Breathe into your heart. Pause. Breathe out. Do this three more times.

- Breathe into your diaphragm, feeling your belly, sacrum, and pelvic floor expand. Breathe out, pulling your scapulae down and towards each other and drawing your navel towards your spine. Do this three more times.

- Move in any way that expresses your fluidity.

2. Relational Field:

- Remember your body does not stop at your skin; imagine a bubble surrounding you and your partner.

- With your eyes closed, feel into the energy in the relational field. What are the qualities (vibrations, energies, size, texture, color, shape, charge, volume, membrane, sound) of this field?

- Blink your eyes open to make brief eye contact with your partner. Close your eyes to notice any changes (breath, heart energy, sensations, vibrations, emotions, impulses). Are there Parts that arise? Do these Parts need anything from you?

- Play with various positions, postures, and distances between you and your partner—engaging with your partner from your front body and back body—to find what best supports you to receive the vibrational energy of your partner.

- Make longer eye contact with your partner. Communicate with your partner using only nonverbal right-brain communication.

- What have you discovered from this exercise about your Self and Parts in relationship?

- Is your impulse to give, receive, or both?

- Share with your partner how you noticed your resonance and what you noticed.

EXPERIENTIAL EXERCISE
RESTORING A RESONANT FLOW

1. Person A thinks of a relationship with a person who activates a Part of them.

2. Person A finds the Part of them that gets activated and notices thoughts, emotions, body sensations, and movement impulses. Then Person A embodies their Part that gets activated by this other person, feeling in their body the activation.

3. Person B mirrors the embodiment of Person A's activated Part.

4. Person A separates from their Part and reestablishes their Embodied Self energy. Person A may use somatic approaches they have learned to restore their Self energy.

5. Person A transmits their Self energy, verbally and nonverbally, to the Part being role-played by Person B until their Part feels seen, understood, and held in compassion by Person A as reported by Person B.

6. Person A thinks again of the relationship with the person who activated their Part and notices what has changed in their inner system.

EXPERIENTIAL EXERCISE
REPAIRING A RELATIONAL RUPTURE

Decide with your partner who will be A (the resonator) and who will be B (the one resonated with). Person A and Person B will role-play a sequence, starting with resonating with each other, experiencing a rupture, and repairing the rupture.

1. Resonance:

- Person B considers how they want to use this time with Person A—share something that is important to them, play, move, etc.

- Person A establishes Self energy; attunes with Person B; makes eye contact; mirror's Person B's movements—anything to express their resonant presence with Person B for several minutes.

- Person B notices what is happening in their body as they feel Person A's resonance and verbally shares their experience with Person A.

2. Rupture:

- In the middle of Person B's sharing, Person A shifts from being present and resonating with Person B to looking away, not responding to Person B, being expressionless, acting distracted or critical. Person A does this for a minute or less.

- Person A restores their Embodied Self energy.

- Person B notices what has shifted in their body and mind.

3. Repair:

- Person A attunes again to Person B and asks Person B to share their internal response to the "rupture."

- Person A resonates with Person B's experience and any Parts that arose.

- Each partner shares what they learned from this role play.

EXPERIENTIAL EXERCISE
GUESS THE BURDEN

1. Person A gets in touch with a Part with a relational burden.

- Person A embodies this burdened Part and invites the Part to express its beliefs, emotions, and behaviors nonverbally—with facial expressions, gestures, posture, sounds, movement.

2. Person B receives the energy and information flowing from Person A.

- Person B resonates with the vibrations of the sensations and emotions.
- Person B mirrors Person A's embodiment with facial expressions, gestures, posture, sounds, movement.
- Person B receives information from the relational field about Person A's Part (age, category of Part, Part's fears, stories, what it needs).

3. Person A appreciates their Part.

4. Person B shares the information they received and the "guesses" they made about Person A's burdened Part.

5. Person A responds.

6. Person A and Person B can switch roles.

EXPERIENTIAL EXERCISE
FOR A SMALL GROUP OR DYAD:
FRONT, MIDDLE, BACK BODY

This exercise was developed by Karby Allington-Goldfain, a staff member for Somatic IFS. Review with the group the fetal development of front, middle, and back body cells, structure, and function.

1. Have the group stand in a circle. Invite one person at a time to stand in the middle with their eyes closed.

2. Ask the group to transmit resonant Self energy from their back body towards the middle of the circle so the person in the middle will feel and experience that energy. People in the circle may want to experiment with first facing towards the center and then turning and having their backs towards the center.

3. Pause and invite the whole group to feel into their body and what they notice.

4. Repeat this with the middle body and front body, experimenting with body position as is appropriate, pausing with each for reflection.

5. When everyone has experienced being in the middle of the circle, share experiences.

Radical Resonance and Collective Trauma

I come as one, but I stand as ten thousand.

—MAYA ANGELOU, "OUR GRANDMOTHERS"

We may have all come on different ships, but we're in the same boat now.

—MARTIN LUTHER KING JR.

> The reality of a quantum universe reunites the Cartesian separation of mind and matter that has dominated Western thought and practices. Quantum physics reunites us with our ancient roots, revealing that matter and energy are completely entangled, leading to a worldview not unlike that of our most ancient ancestors and some still surviving indigenous cultures who believe that rocks, water, air, and animals—including humans—are all equally imbued with spirit, with invisible energy.[1]

We can apply Radical Resonance to every level of the body system. We consider the quantum, molecular, and cellular levels and the individual body and its physical systems involved in our resonant capacity. We also consider the role of social systems in our relational lives—various social identities, cultures, and institutions, and even the planetary and cosmic levels. We recognize the entangled reciprocal relationships between all these levels of systems. Cultural burdens affect individuals, and unburdened individuals can affect societal and institutional burdens.

The origin of the adjective *radical* is *root*. As Marcus Garvey once wrote, "A people without knowledge of their past history, origin and culture is like a tree without roots." We reach into our roots as we now shift our focus from exploring intrapersonal and interpersonal resonant relationships to our resonance with intergenerational, ancestral, and community relationships. Just as our bodies hold stories and histories from our personal lives from conception to the present day, they also carry stories from our ancestors—our parents, grandparents, great grandparents, and other relatives, even from earlier centuries. We carry both the gifts and the trauma in our bodies.

Many of our ancestors may have experienced trauma from war, torture, poverty, and famine. The repercussions of their wounds persist beyond their lives and can be found in the bodies and lives of those that follow. The wounds that were not able to be processed were handed on to us, like broken antique furniture. Those burdens of the direct survivors of the traumatic or devaluing events were passed on through their DNA, stories, and behaviors. We call these "legacy burdens" in IFS. The actual events may take different shapes and forms from generation to generation. Ancestral Unburdening is a gift for us as individuals, for our ancestors, and for future generations.

EXPERIENTIAL EXERCISE
RESONATING WITH OUR ANCESTORS

1. Begin by establishing your inner vertical alignment. Check in with your inner system for any activation as you explore your ancestral roots.

2. Name and describe your ancestral roots: racial, cultural, national, ethnic, language, class, and so on.

3. What information do you have about your ancestors? Do you know of verbal or written stories or legends about your ancestors?

4. What do you know or imagine happened to your ancestors that needed to be exiled, frozen in their bodies and minds, so that they could survive?

5. What gifts do you attribute to your ancestral heritage?

6. What burdens do you attribute to your ancestral heritage?

7. How does your body carry these gifts and burdens?

HEALING ANCESTRAL BURDENS

Our everyday, largely unconscious movements may have originated in the traumatic experiences of our parents, grandparents, or even ancient ancestors through bodily inheritance and culturally defining experiences. Just as bringing awareness to our sensations and breathing can reveal the implicitly held memories of our earliest experiences, they can lead us to our legacy burdens, allowing a release of the burden stored in our cells, nervous systems, and muscles and fascia, and ending the cycle of unprocessed trauma carried through the generations.

Ciara McGriskin, a participant in my Somatic IFS programs and founder of Souliology, which organizes my SIFS programs, shares her experience and an exercise to assist you in working with your ancestral burdens.

> I've delved into my ancestral line, specifically connecting with my father's maternal lineage. The deep connection extends to Norse healers from distant ancestry who endured persecution during the Christian era. Their pagan way of life, deemed unacceptable, forced them to conceal their beliefs and traditions for survival. This resonated profoundly with me, as in my present life, my Parts always carried a sense of needing to hide and sense of not belonging, and I wasn't fully clear where this came from.

Engaging with them and aiding in the release of their burdens—stemming from nonacceptance and a sense of not belonging—has been transformative. This process also liberated me from the burden of concealing my beliefs, fostering a commitment to intertwine our healing gifts into my daily life and work. The experience has bolstered my self-belief. It has helped foster a profound connection to the earth and Mother Nature, and it has led me to a strong sense of alignment with the inherent qualities of my ancestors.

I am consistently shedding the fear of standing behind my beliefs, which has given me the courage to guide myself and my family to embrace what feels right and natural to us, even if it diverges from conventional beliefs. The Ancestral Unburdening process has had an indelible impact on my life and has opened the door to daily connection with them. It has also helped shift my ultimate life goal to carry forward the much needed work that they were barred from undertaking and sharing.

EXPERIENTIAL EXERCISE
ANCESTRAL UNBURDENING

By Ciara McGriskin

1. You may have found a burdened belief, emotion, sensation, or behavior that you sense is not connected with your personal experience in your life but is influencing your present life in significant ways. You might experience this ancestral burden as a physical, psychological, or energy block, or like a piece of yourself is missing—put away for *safekeeping* by your Ancestors in times of trauma, chaos, or difficult challenges.

2. Allow all the time your body needs to connect securely with the ground below; root your energy and awareness more deeply into the earth that holds the bones of your ancestors.

3. Gently and mindfully bring your attention to where and how you are carrying this burden in your body, asking your system to show you the source of this burden.

4. As you bring awareness to this burden, consider your lineage on both of your parents' sides. Which one are you most drawn to explore? Which ancestral line feels like it might also have carried this burden? You may have a sense you are connecting with a specific ancestor, or you might more generally connect with some situation that impacted your ancestors.

5. There may be a movement, touch, or words that can communicate your Self energy to your ancestors, and to the place in your body where you are holding this burden or block.

6. Notice any images, emotions, thoughts, words, sensations, or movement impulses that come to you. Stay with the energy and information coming to you and allow it to unfold. You might want to draw the image or record the words or thoughts.

7. Ask the ancestor to help you understand what was happening at the time they took on this burden. You can ask them to show you what happened. They can tell you, show you a memory or an image, point to a historical event, or point to an unhealthy cultural belief. Ask them:

   • Why did they feel they needed to take on this burden?

   • What was it like for them to carry this burden?

   • What, if any, were the benefits from taking on this burden?

   • How did it help them?

   • Were there any heirlooms to carrying this burden? Invite it and welcome it in whatever form it comes to you.

   • Does this ancestor recognize you? How would you describe your relationship?

8. You can offer to help the ancestor release the burden in any way that feels right to them. Free the burden all along the ancestral line from its source in history to you in present time. As you help the ancestor to fully release the burden, you can let them know you are also helping to release all future generations, both known and unknown, from having to continue to carry the burden.

9. After the unburdening, the ancestor may need some reassurance, forgiveness, and appreciation that they did what they had to do to survive. You can help the ancestor restore any qualities lost as a result of their trauma.

10. When this feels complete, say goodbye, and then check with your own system to see if there are Parts that may need further assistance as a result of carrying this ancestral burden.

The backdrop to our ancestral stories and trauma stories lies in our cultural burdens. These burdens can be found in our bodies as well as in our body politic, in the basic fabric of society and its institutions—in our economic, legal, penal, educational, military, and religious systems. We have been born into a collectively traumatized world where the basic assumption is separation.

Our Western culture's dualistic and hierarchical separation of mind and body can be seen to be at the root of our cultural burdens of polarization, fragmentation, isolation, and dominance. We have inherited and been formed by a culture that is racist, patriarchal, capitalist, and materialist. A culture that idealizes White bodies, male bodies, cisgendered bodies, heterosexual bodies, nondisabled bodies. A culture that rewards cognition, competition, production, and verbal and written communication. A culture that fosters meritocracy, individualism, separateness, and scarcity. A culture that systematically and systemically exiles, objectifies, exploits, and oppresses women, people of color, and vulnerable populations with life-threatening inequities. Many of us are hungry for a sense of belonging after generations of disconnection, displacement, colonialism, and oppression. The legacy burdens from our culture hold us hostage in a cycle of shame, blame, and self-criticism, blocking our capacity for resonance and our fullest embodiment.

EMBODIED SOCIAL IDENTITY

In the chart below, there are eight categories related to bodily appearance and functioning.

The three descriptions of each category show the sociocultural groups from most devalued, oppressed, and marginalized at left to most valued and associated with power and privilege at right.

Our assigned membership in sociocultural groups, according to physical traits that are considered desirable or deficient, affects every aspect of our lives. Although some of us are deemed winners and others losers, we all, in fact, lose as we are cut off from our bodies and from each other. When our bodies and identities are not valued by the dominant culture, many of us do not value our bodies. We judge them, neglect them, objectify them, punish them, and exile them. For survival, our protective Parts may mimic what is valued and reject what is devalued in ourselves and others. What has been exiled is not lost, but is stored in our bodies and the collective body waiting for compassionate witnessing to rise to the surface and be known and redeemed.

CATEGORY	DEVALUED		VALUED
body size	large	average	slim
language	non-English	learned English	English
gender	trans, intersex, nonbinary	cisgender woman	cisgender man
skin color	dark	different shades	white
ability or disability	significant disability	some disability	nondisabled
sexuality	lesbian, bi, pan, asexual	gay men	heterosexual
neurodiversity	significant neurodivergence	neuroatypical	neurotypical
age	very young, older person	middle-aged	young adult

Adapted from Canadian Council for Refugees, "Wheel of Power and Privilege," https://ccrweb.ca.

1. Consider your body appearance and function with each category:

   - body size
   - language
   - gender
   - skin color

   - ability or disability
   - sexuality
   - neurodiversity
   - age

2. Are there categories of embodied social identity not mentioned in the chart above that you want to consider, such as marital status, immigration status, parenting status, religion, educational level, citizenship? If so, include them in the three-part sequence of social valuation.

CATEGORY	DEVALUED		VALUED

3. What Parts arise as you consider these socially constructed valuations? Take time with each of these Parts, befriending them and listening to them verbally and nonverbally.

_____

_____

_____

4. Name your identities that have been **valued** by your culture (right column).

_____

_____

_____

- How have you experienced the privileges and advantages of each one?

  _____

  _____

  _____

- What Parts arise as you consider your privileged status?

  _____

  _____

  _____

- What do your protector Parts fear if you were to lose your privilege?

  _____

  _____

  _____

- What are the behaviors of the Parts?

  _____

  _____

  _____

- How do your Parts perceive others who do not share this identity?

  _____

  _____

  _____

- What has been exiled to maintain your privileged status?

  _____

  _____

  _____

5. Name your identities that have been **devalued** by your culture (two left columns).

_____

_____

_____

- Consider the protector Parts' burdens.

  _____

  _____

  _____

- How do your Parts perceive others who do not share this identity?

  _____

  _____

  _____

- What have you had to exile because it was devalued?

  _____

  _____

  _____

- Find your burdened vulnerable Parts and bring your compassion to them.

  _____

  _____

  _____

- Can you help your Parts let go of their burden of individual blame and shame? Let them feel your resonance with their burdens, and use any of the Somatic IFS practices.

  _____

  _____

  _____

6. Which category of your identity has been the most impactful in your life?

_____

_____

_____

- Embody the Part or Parts that arise. What burdens do they carry?

  _____

  _____

  _____

- Resonate with them; witness their story.

  _____

  _____

  _____

Remember, our social identities are evident in our bodies. Before we have language, we learn about our social group and how to survive in them (our families, communities, and so on). Our habitual movements, gaits, and gestures reflect our attempts to survive in a culture built on exercising power over others and nature, and they communicate those attempts to the external world. The survival-oriented autonomic nervous systems we have inherited dictate whether we puff ourselves up to fight, turn away to flee, collapse, hunker down to endure, or signal appeasement.

EXPERIENTIAL EXERCISE
EMBODYING YOUR SOCIAL IDENTITY

1. What behaviors, gestures, and stances do you associate with each of your identities?

2. In what ways have your social identities deemed valuable affected how you feel towards your body?

3. In what ways have your marginalized and devalued social identities affected how you feel towards your body?

4. In what ways have your social identities deemed valuable affected your body behaviors?

5. In what ways have your marginalized and devalued social identities affected your body behaviors?

6. In what ways have cultural valuations and devaluations affected your relationships?

Releasing Collective Burdens in Small Groups

As we restore our resonant capacities and become more embodied, we are beginning to dissolve the cultural burdens of separation, polarization, and fragmentation for ourselves, those who came before us, and those yet to come. Those of us whose social identities are associated with power and privilege need to unlearn embodied patterns that keep oppression in place. For example, as those of us with White American bodies face the pain that the land we claim is soaked with the blood of Indigenous people, and that our privileged status rests on the backs of enslaved African people owned by our ancestors, we begin to heal the split in ourselves and the world around us. As Ken Hardy says, it starts with gut-wrenching courage to resonate with another's pain, and to stay long enough to allow something to emerge that can be healed:

> White people must be willing to break their silence regarding whiteness and its long-term, pervasive, and deleterious effects on the lives of People of Color and all of humanity. White people must be forthright and engage in a gut-wrenching truth-telling about their whiteness, their complicity with the centrality of whiteness, and what they pledge regarding dismantling the prevailing racial order.[2]

We can break out of our individualistic patterns. Collective burdens need a collective to heal. Affiliating with those who share aspects of our social identities, we notice, name, and unburden Parts associated with that identity. By connecting with our ancestors and elders, we form the rooted, radical bond for embodied transformation. Collectively, we may be inspired to also consider actions to deconstruct the inequities of the institutional structures that injure the souls of all people.

In no way does this lessen that our ancestors' legacies also include many blessings. Along with burdens, we have inherited from our loving and wise ancestors many collective somatic practices to bring the body out of exile from our individual and societal wounds, to restore and cultivate our body's awareness, sensitivities, and responsivity. Their blessings open a pathway to connect with our roots and transform our inherited burdens. Tapping into the wellspring of ancestral support, we can heal the body-mind split individually and societally. We turn to our ancestors to embody the strengths and blessings of our unique, diverse bloodlines.

The collective practices include humming, sounding, singing, chanting, drumming; rituals, ceremonies, prayers, dream work, movement; connecting with the four elements, energies, and spirits from the four directions.

EXPERIENTIAL EXERCISE
SMALL GROUP—BRINGING COLLECTIVE PRACTICES TO CULTURAL BURDENS

1. Gather a small group of people who share most of your social identities and are willing to meet over time.

2. Use Somatic IFS to develop safety and trust.

3. Each group member speaks for their protector Parts, addressing their fears, helping them unblend until there is sufficient Self energy available to support this work.

4. The group expresses this collective Self energy through movement, sound, or any other form of expression.

5. One group member selects a Part to focus on that has absorbed burdens inherited from their culture. They—with guidance and support from group members—embody the selected Part. Other group members may mirror the Part, resonate with it, and bring compassion to the Part through movement, sound, drumming, or ritual.

6. The group member stays with their Part, inviting it to let go of its cultural burdens.

7. Each group member shares their experience of the collective practice.

8. Another group member chooses a Part with a cultural burden to experience collective resonance.

EXPERIENTIAL EXERCISE
SMALL GROUP RESONANCE

1. Person A verbally and nonverbally shares a cultural burden with the group for a set time (about fifteen minutes).

2. Each person in the group takes on a role during Person A's sharing:

   - Tracking Person A's body: breath, movement, touch.
   - Tracking their own body: sensations, breath, movement, touch.
   - Tracking their own emotions, images, thoughts, memories.
   - Opening to messages from their ancestors, the larger Field of Self energy, and their guides. If there are more than five people, several people can take this role.

3. Each person shares what they noticed while listening to Person A.

4. Person A shares their response to hearing from the other group members.

5. Rotate the roles so everyone gets a turn to share a cultural burden.

Clinical Application of Radical Resonance
The 3 R's: Receptivity, Resonance, Revision

Although the language for this part of the chapter will be "therapist" and "client," much of this information about the therapeutic relationship is applicable to any important relationship—with a child or other family member, a spouse or partner, friends, and colleagues.

We have learned from neuroscientific research about neural plasticity and that we are inherently hardwired to make somatic shifts in relation to another person. With this understanding, therapists see the importance of psychobiological attunement with the client, and that their body is the vehicle for this. A Somatic IFS therapist receives the client's verbal stories while the untold, unconscious, implicit story is being communicated nonverbally to the receptive right brain and body of the therapist. The therapist's body reverberates with the vibrational frequencies of the client's voiced and unvoiced painful experiences. The therapist synchronizes with the client's state, transmitting their Self energy to the client, verbally and nonverbally. The frequencies of the burdened Parts of the client are brought into coherence with the frequency of Self energy.

While writing these words, struggling to convey this practice with these academic left-brain concepts, Beth ONeil, a previously mentioned Somatic IFS therapist and staff member (and also my wife), emerged from her office after a virtual session with a client. She shared how she resonated with her client's responsible, caretaking protector Parts. Her resonating Parts did not take over. The resonance helped her feel more intimately connected. She said it was because she was mostly able to stay in Self. Her Parts resonated, as did her Self, expanding her view of her client's entire internal system. Beth's Self energy may have been transmitted to her client, because then her client deepened into a somatic experience of the exile that had been pushed down by her protectors. I asked Beth how she noticed that in her body. At first, it was not easy for her to describe, and I could resonate with the struggle to find the words. But together we identified a few metaphors—like when the sun pops out and illuminates the path—and a sudden energetic shift that awakens our senses to a new level. Beth stroked her front torso, and her spine lengthened. As she continued to reflect on the session, she said she thought the shift to deepen happened in her seconds before it did in her client.

> Rather than being an observer or even an experienced guide, the therapist reverberates with the tremors of abuse, neglect, betrayal, and abandonment. The Parts' tacit stories feel fathomed. Their burdened beliefs about rejection and isolation dissolve in the emotional, right-brain watery relational realm. . . . The resulting energies are more than an additive process, greater than transmission or contagion. The dynamic interplay cocreated within the relational field multiplies the Embodied Self energy exponentially. . . . If most of the energy exchange in our therapy offices is below the level of our awareness, we can begin by being aware that we are not aware of it. With intention and receptivity, our ability to sense energy transmissions can develop.[3]

Developing Our Resonance and Receptivity

For clients to get the visceral experience of being safely held for their physiology to calm down, heal, and grow, they need our bodies to be a clear vessel, like a singing bowl that resonates with the client. We would like to be that for others at all times, but it is not always possible. We all have been hurt in many relationships, and we carry the scars, many of them unconscious, into all our relationships. Our Parts continue to try to protect us from being humiliated, rejected, blamed, or sucked into another's trauma vortex. Being a therapist (or a parent, spouse, or friend) is risky business.

In order to safely resonate, to be open to receiving another's experience without getting lost in it or reacting to it, we need to be able to access our Self energy. When in Embodied Self, we are in the state of *being with* rather than *doing to*. Our Self-like protector Parts that believe they have to make correct and even brilliant interpretations relax. We stay open to the moment-by-moment flow of energy between the client and ourselves. Instead of leaving awareness of our own bodymind system aside while we focus on our clients, especially their narrative, we find a balance of attention of self and other. We listen internally to our Parts' thoughts, our bodies, our emotions, and any information that may be coming to us from the Field of Self energy.

We can also experiment with making a few changes to our habitual ways of relating. Some Somatic IFS therapists have found that they typically tune in to their front bodies when engaged with a client, and then when they intentionally tune into their back bodies instead, they find it easier to resonate with the pain, shame, and fear of their clients. Others have found that tuning into the fluidity of their body helps with Parts that need to know, allowing them to flow with the tides and rhythms of the client's process. I have heard from Somatic IFS therapists that they enjoy therapy more. Their clients don't just feel understood; they feel "felt." They are more able to resonate with their own Parts. Their Self becomes the agent of healing their wounds of abandonment and abuse, providing secure attachment to their Parts.

EXPERIENTIAL EXERCISE
REFLECTING ON RESONANCE IN A SESSION

In addition to, or instead of, taking notes on your client's experience, jot down what you notice happening in your body and mind while being with the client, either during the session or immediately afterwards.

1. How did you establish your Embodied Self energy?

2. What in your body let you know you were in Self energy?

3. Were there moments during the session when it was more challenging to stay in Self?

4. How did you establish the relational bubble?

5. Did you connect with your client mostly from your front body or back body?

6. What was most helpful for your resonance—considering the solid, spacious, or fluid nature of your body?

7. Which of your resonant organs did you intentionally engage: limbic brain, heart, gut?

8. What were some of your internal responses during the session?

- Emotions:
- Sensations:
- Breath:

- Movement impulses from any part of your body:

- Thoughts:

9. We usually assume our internal responses are ours. Could any of them have been transmitted energetically and vibrationally from your client's system?

10. Neuroscientists tell us that resonance is a mutual process, rewiring the therapist's inner system as well as the client's. Did you experience anything that indicates a shift in your inner system?

11. How was it for you to focus more on your own experience? In what ways do you think it impacted this session?

From Receptivity to Revision: Shifts Happen

Resonance can repair and reshape the neural firing patterns in the client's brain and revise other chemical and energetic patterns in the body damaged by trauma and faulty attachment from conception to the present, as well as from intergenerational and transgenerational traumas. Neural revision is a right brain-to-right brain process, and it is mutual. The changes are throughout the body, including the brains of both therapist and client.

Unburdening is only one of the many transformations that can happen during the course of a therapy session. The shifts may seem subtle—easy to miss or gloss over—especially if the therapist is reluctant to ask the client to stop their narrating or reporting in order to pause long enough to notice the change. The resonant therapist tracks for any shifts that are happening for the client, any new and unfamiliar experiences. The therapist invites a pause of several breaths to notice and appreciate the change. During these seconds of pausing, the new positive experience registers in the brain. The neuronal bonds of the client's habitual burden-informed wiring are weakening. New synaptic bonds are forming. As the new experience is encouraged and practiced over time, the synaptic bonds will strengthen from repeated firings, creating new neural circuitries, pathways, and networks that support healthy, resilient relationships.

EXPERIENTIAL EXERCISE
NOTICING, NAMING, SAVORING THE POSITIVE SHIFTS

1. Ask a client if they would be interested in you carefully tracking their process as it unfolds in order to appreciate the changes, even the subtle ones, that indicate positive shifts in their inner system. Let the client know you will be asking them to pause for a few breaths when you notice that something has shifted.

2. You might explain to the client that the pause and the moment to appreciate and savor allow for the growth of new neural circuits of trust, compassion, and curiosity. Invite the client to also notice their changes and choose to pause.

_____

_____

_____

3. Some examples of shifts the client may experience:

- Sensing the therapist's full-bodied listening.
- Discovering a Part that had been locked away.
- The protector trusts Self energy and can relax.
- The Part is no longer isolated.
- Increased awareness of sensation.
- Ability to take a deeper breath.
- Release of tension or holding anywhere in the body.
- Speech is more embodied.
- Protector Parts feeling appreciated rather than demonized.
- Spontaneous unburdenings.
- Relational shifts in Parts' interrelationships.
- Any of the ways that Embodied Self impacts the internal system.

4. Shifts noticed and named:

_____

_____

_____

5. Client's experience after the pause.

Most therapists will encounter some habitual patterns with these 3 R's: receptivity resonance, and revision. Check the ones you have noticed:

❑ I have difficulty feeling into the relational field.

❑ I too easily resonate with my client's Parts and become flooded by their emotional states.

❑ I am afraid I will lose myself in the relationship.

❑ I am afraid my own unhealed attachment wounds will be activated.

  ❏ I don't experience this right-brain communication.

  ❏ I rely primarily on left-brain therapeutic interventions.

  ❏ My protector Parts use emotional distancing for the needed boundaries.

  ❏ I am afraid of being overwhelmed by my client's somatic and emotional experiences.

  ❏ I am reluctant to direct my client to pause to notice the shifts in their system. I don't want to interrupt their process.

  ❏ I am not sure that I have healed enough of my own attachment wounds to be able to stay in Self energy.

  ❏ Other:

_____

_____

_____

EXPERIENTIAL EXERCISE
ADDRESSING YOUR PARTS' CONCERNS

1. Choose one of the statements above to explore with Somatic IFS.

2. As you consider the statement, how and where does it land in your body?

3. Although some of them are "I" statements, a Part is speaking. How do you feel towards the Part?

4. What does the Part want you to know about its fears, habits, or difficulties?

5. What does the Part need from you to trust your receptivity and resonance to allow for reciprocal revision?

Receptivity, Resonance, and Revision with Attachment Wounds

Our current intimate relationships may reveal Parts burdened by our earliest relational experiences. Beginning in the womb, our early attachment experiences are transmitted as vibrational frequencies via our bodies and right-brain structures. We receive frequencies from both the Parts and Self of our caregivers. These roots of our early relational lives are recorded subcortically. They are mostly nonverbal. These deep, hidden roots impact our relationships in myriad ways.

As Somatic IFS practices bring these early experiences to our awareness, these very young traumatized Parts communicate with us largely through right-brain language—facial expressions, gestures, emotions, movements, sounds, visual images, touch, taste. We receive their nonverbal right-brain communication and resonate with it.

> The client's own Embodied Self energy emerges as the secure attachment figure for the client's young Parts. The vibrations of Embodied Self energy in both therapist and client are amplified. The resulting energies are more than an additive process, greater than transmission or contagion. The dynamic interplay cocreated within the relational field multiplies the Embodied Self energy exponentially.[4]

The therapist receives the verbal and nonverbal messages and resonates with the burdens—the emotions, sensations, and behaviors. The therapist identifies the type of insecure attachment and brings all the qualities of Self energy so the client can have a new, healthy relational experience.

- Insecure-avoidant attachment style: Parts have difficulty with trust, emotional expression, closeness, conflict.

- Insecure-anxious: Parts are clingy, needy for reassurance, overly dependent, fearful of abandonment.

- Disorganized: Parts are volatile and polarized in regard to intimacy, feeling unworthy of love.

WHAT THE THERAPIST CAN SAY TO FACILITATE A RESONANT RELATIONSHIP

- "What is happening in your body as you tell me this?"

- "How is it for you to experience this with me?"

- "I am touched that you shared that with me."

- "What do you see in my eyes as I am feeling this with you?"

- "You are not alone. I am here with you."

- "I noticed you turned away when I said that. Let's stay with this to get to know that Part."

- "What does your Part need from me right now?"

- "Can we find objects in the room to represent each of your Parts?"

- "How does this Part feel towards you? How can you help it?"

Integration of Radical Resonance

Perhaps resonance takes us to where the ideas of therapist and client, self and other begin to dissolve, expanding beyond interpersonal, intrapersonal, and transpersonal healing to establish a more harmonious relationship with other human beings, with all living beings, with the planet, even with the universe. Perhaps restoring our ability to resonate could heal our narcissistic Parts' view that we have the right to dominate other people, animals, earth. Maybe it could result in more social and economic equality. Instead of continuing our practice of controlling earth's resources for our own gain, we could avoid the sixth mass extinction where over a million species will disappear from the planet. Perhaps this dream begins with the courage to radically resonate with another's pain.[5]

With this chapter, we stepped into the horizontal relational realm to explore how somatic practices and IFS can assist us with the complexity as inner systems interact. We explored Radical Resonance with another person, collectively and intergenerationally, and with our clients. We experienced our inherent capacity to resonate. Additionally, we understand that we are hardwired to take in the energies and the vibrational frequencies of others' Parts as well as the Self energy of others.

We all know what happens when we interact with a partner, friend, parent, or child who is blended with their burdened Parts and we cannot sustain our Self energy. Our resonant capacity activates our own Parts, and we find ourselves in an escalating Parts skirmish. If we can stay curious, calm, and maybe even compassionate, we can deepen our relationship. We are familiar with our default Parts-led relational patterns based on our own relational experiences. We may react, confront, and defend, or we may distance, detach, and avoid. We also understand the healing potential of Self-led resonance to repair our relational wounds and enhance our relationships.

This chapter has acquainted you with several ways to help you repair and maintain your resonant capacity. We may find it helpful to shift our focus from our front bodies to our middle or back bodies, or our balance of attention between self and other. We may tune into the fluid nature of our bodies and tend to our heart, gut, and right brain communication. We may open to energy, information, and guidance from the Self Field and ancestors. In these ways, we have entered the rich territory of interpersonal relationships where the frequencies of our Embodied Self energy can repair and revise the bodymind systems of others. We are ready to consider the benefits of movement as a potent source of nonverbal communication in our relationships for healing individual and societal burdens.

Take some moments to reflect on all you have absorbed from this chapter, the readings, exercises, and your own responses and questions.

1. What exercises or information did you find most helpful, useful, or relevant?

_____

_____

_____

2. What do you most want to remember to be able to practice and develop in your own way?

_____

_____

_____

3. Is there anything about interpersonal resonance that you want to explore further on this topic?

_____

_____

_____

4. Did any information or exercises feel confusing, irrelevant, or too activating?

_____

_____

_____

5. Have you experienced any shifts you want to celebrate, savor, and anchor?

_____

_____

_____

Notes

1 Susan McConnell, *Somatic Internal Family Systems Therapy*, 132.

2 Kenneth V. Hardy, preface to *The Enduring, Invisible, and Ubiquitous Centrality of Whiteness* (New York: W. W. Norton, 2022).

3 Susan McConnell, *Somatic Internal Family Systems Therapy*, 131–32.

4 Susan McConnell, *Somatic Internal Family Systems Therapy*, 131.

5 Susan McConnell, *Somatic Internal Family Systems Therapy*, 134.

5

Mindful Movement

Purpose of Mindful Movement

HAVING ESTABLISHED A FOUNDATION of an embodied relationship with earth and sky with the Somatic IFS practices of awareness and breath, and having moved into the horizontal plane where we can experience resonant relationships, we explore the practice of Mindful Movement as it relates to the IFS Model and other forms of somatic therapies.

This practice includes bringing mindfulness to our habitual movement patterns that, like Somatic Awareness and Conscious Breathing, are the outward manifestations of our inner worlds. Compassionate, curious exploration of these movements or restricted movement impulses welcomes the untold traumatic stories embedded in the tissues to unfold, offering a path for restoring the flow.

Movement is inextricably linked to our intentions, beliefs, needs, and desires. It is at the heart of our social interactions, celebrations, and cultural expressions. Movement, both spontaneous and directed, can be a source of joy, stress relief, fun, and creative expression, and it contributes to our physical and emotional well-being. Movement practices *can* support and sustain Embodied Self energy.

Individual Application of Mindful Movement

Movement is the primal language of our emotions. Our Parts' emotions want to be expressed and acknowledged. The Latin root of the word *emotions* is *emovere,* meaning "to move out." Our protectors, believing they need to bury the potentially overwhelming emotions of the vulnerable Parts, control and contain our movements. Our image managers may have learned to inhibit socially unacceptable movements. Yet our emotions look for a way to move out. Bringing mindfulness to our spontaneous movements and dormant impulses to move can safely allow the movement stories to be told, restoring the flow of our emotions and life force.

We bring mindful awareness to movements gross and subtle, habitual and interrupted, conscious and unconscious. We notice facial movements like smiles, sneers, clenched teeth and jaws, raised or furrowed eyebrows, and eye movements. Heads may reach, shake, cock, turn away, nod, hang down. Hands may clutch, grip, push, go flaccid. Feet may shuffle, tap, wiggle, cross. The torso may collapse or puff up. Shoulders may shrug, curl in, or lift up.

All of these gestures, postures, and more often accompany the verbal story. Mindfulness of these movements signals a welcome invitation to a Part's story. The story, whether acquired, inherited, or energetically transmitted intergenerationally, can be expressed through movement and witnessed by Embodied Self.

The movement story may be one of trauma, sequencing from the first attempts to orient to find safety, then the adaptive reflexes to fight or flee, the collapse when the body's resources are overwhelmed, and finally the trembling that signals a release of the pent-up energies.

Movement may tell of our earliest attempts to reach out, push away, cling, or move towards what we longed for. If those attempts were thwarted, they may have led to burdens of shame, fear, and disappointment as well as disruptions in our cognitive and social development. These early movement experiences are evident in our lifelong movement patterns. Reenacting these movements allows the frozen impulses and associated emotions to sequence through the body.

Our protector Parts may have adopted movements or lack of movement to protect the system. Mindfulness of the movements is key to avoiding a cathartic retraumatization. Mindfulness creates the conditions for Embodied Self energy to witness, digest, and integrate the stories of unresolved trauma or interrupted motor development. These stories—frozen for years in faces, repetitive gestures, and chronic pain and stiffness—thaw in the warmth of Mindful Movement. We welcome, witness, and transform our burdened Parts, freeing up our Embodied Self energy. When the flow is restored, the dance of our inner systems is harmonious, creative, and life-giving.

EXPERIENTIAL EXERCISE
YOUR INNER DANCE

1. Sitting: Notice the rhythmic pulsations of breath and heart, digestion, muscles tightening or letting go, slight shifts in alignment.

2. Welcome your inner dance. It might begin with stillness, lying down, or moving through space. Let one movement give rise to the next. If your movements are similar to your habitual movements, or if they begin to feel repetitive, try a new movement.

3. Are there places in your body that would like to move more fully? If so, follow that impulse.

   • Does the movement lead you to an emotion? To a Part? To Self energy?

   • Does the movement tell a story?

4. Are there places in your body that don't want to move or don't move freely?

   • Bring your focused attention to these places.

- What do you learn about these places that don't move freely? Do you find a Part? If so, how do you feel towards this Part?

- Is the Part willing to let you play with movement (perhaps subtle, slight, slow movement)? If not, what are its fears? If so, what happens as you play with a movement in this part of your body?

5. Which movements felt enjoyable? Which movements felt uncomfortable or impossible?

6. Complete your inner dance with a movement that expresses your acceptance of yourself just as you are.

SAFETY GUIDELINES

Track your sensations, breath, heart, and gut to gauge your level of activation. Use any tools you learned in the last three chapters to return safety and calm to your inner system.

Feel free to pause or skip any exercise.

EXPERIENTIAL EXERCISE
EARLY MOVEMENT MEMORIES

As discussed, our burdened Parts influence our movements. Some of our Parts suppress or contain movement, while others may use movement for achieving, performing, and competing. Both of these Parts can affect our mental and physical well-being. We can find those Parts as we consider our earliest memories of moving:

1. Your first memory of moving.

2. Times you mastered or succeeded at a movement.

3. Types of movement that were a challenge, where you felt inadequate.

4. Accidents or injuries that resulted from movements.

5. Movements that were restricted or judged.

6. Movements that brought you pleasure and enjoyment.

7. What burdened beliefs, emotions, and behaviors do your Parts carry today as a result of your movement history?

8. How has your movement history impacted your current relationship with movement?

Fire Element

The element for Mindful Movement is fire. Like movement, fire is transformative. Fire represents energy, assertiveness, passion, heat, light, and purification. Fire has been a part of rituals for millennia. We release our burdens into the fire where they are transformed into ash and smoke. Movement requires more metabolic fire. The controlled slow burn of metabolism fuels us to thaw out, express and transform our Parts' burdened emotions and behaviors, and move forward in our lives.

EXPERIENTIAL EXERCISE
MOVEMENT TO AWAKEN YOUR INTERNAL FIRE

1. Standing, scan your body for any muscle tension other than what is required for you to stand. Move these muscles until they can relax and rest, making more of your internal fire available.

2. Scan your body for any areas that are numb or outside your awareness. Move these areas until they are more awakened.

3. Check in with your thoughts and emotions. If you feel any stress or anxiety, invite these thoughts and feelings to express themselves in movement until you feel calmer.

4. If your Parts are now able to relax, you will be able to feel Self energy being released in your body.

5. The solar plexus, between the navel and the diaphragm, is the chakra that governs the fire element. This third chakra is your inner power, strength, and vitality, your confidence and self-esteem. Breathe into this place. Feel the rhythmic movement with your hand. Do you feel Self energy flowing through your central channel?

6. How might the energy from this chakra and your central channel want to move your body?

7. Come to rest and stillness as you keep your focus on your solar plexus.

8. Can accessing this fire energy through your solar plexus and central channel assist you as you move towards your life goals?

Our Internal System and Movement

Remember, our Parts communicate their burdens to us, largely outside our awareness, through our habitual gestures, gait, and postures. Movement may be the best, or the only, way for Parts to let us know of the load they are carrying. These movements not only reveal the burdens but reinforce them.

Through our movements, movement impulses, and suppressed movements, we access a somatic record of our Parts' burdened beliefs, emotions, and thoughts. When unburdened, the Parts are freed to use movement in beneficial ways.

- **Manager Parts** use movements or suppress our movement impulses to keep our vulnerable Parts and firefighter Parts contained or controlled. They may use movements to gain social acceptance and perform their protective roles. Unburdened managers may use movement for health and wellness, service, nurturance, and effective action.

- **Firefighter Parts** use movements in two main ways. Movement or suppressed movement is used to soothe, numb, or freeze. They also have impulses to kick, hit, run, recoil, push, and grab and may act them out. Unburdened firefighter Parts may use movement for enjoyment, adventure, and passion, and for standing up to injustice.

- **Vulnerable Parts (exiles)** may tell their stories through movement or immobility. They use movement to express their feelings of helplessness, isolation, unworthiness, shame, fear. Their movement patterns may reveal unresolved trauma, insecure attachment, or interrupted motor development. Unburdened vulnerable Parts may express their tenderness, playfulness, creativity, and innocence through movement.

- **Self:** Movement flows through the body in a balanced, coordinated way expressing the qualities of Self, among them courage, connection, confidence, calmness, curiosity, and compassion.

EXPERIENTIAL EXERCISE
OUR MOVING PARTS

1. Invite one of your manager Parts to come more fully into your awareness.

2. What role does this Part play in your system? What are its concerns if it were not to do this?

3. Let this manager Part show itself to you in your body. Take on the posture, facial expression, and gestures of your hands and arms. Walk through space from this Part's energies and impulses.

4. Mindfully play with one of the manager's movements. Repeat it, slow it down. Exaggerate the movement. Make the movement smaller, more subtle.

5. Are there words, feelings, or images that go with this movement?

6. Did you notice any movements that were blocked or suppressed by a manager Part?

7. Do the same with a firefighter Part and a vulnerable Part.

8. Thank your Parts for being willing to be known in these ways. Is there a movement that can let each Part know you are glad to get to know them more fully? A movement to help them to feel safer and more content and loved?

9. Invite your Parts to join you in a Self-led dance of mutual connection and compassion.

EXPERIENTIAL EXERCISE
MOVEMENT TO FIND, FOCUS, FLESH OUT A PART

As our every thought and emotion is accompanied by a muscular response, our habitual movement patterns, largely outside our awareness, may lead us to a Part with an untold movement story. Consider a movement that you tend to make somewhat automatically or habitually. It might be a gesture, a shift in posture or position, or a way you move through space that is your own signature movement. Choose a movement that you are curious about to find out whether it leads to a Part's story.

1. What movement do you want to explore?

2. How do you feel towards this movement?

3. Just as you did with the previous exercise, play with this movement—make it larger, smaller, slower, faster. Move in a way that would be the opposite of this movement.

4. As you mindfully repeat this movement, are there words, thoughts, emotions, or images that seem connected with it?

5. Does this familiar movement lead you to a Part?

6. Invite this Part to show you or tell you all it wants you to know.

7. Repeat the original movement. Does it change?

Mindful Movement and Trauma

Our movement patterns mediated by burdened Parts can be the result of unprocessed trauma. Our ANS governs how we move through the world, whether we move towards or away from, or whether we freeze, appease, or collapse. With Stephen Porges's pioneering polyvagal theory, we understand that these movement patterns are instinctual and adaptive trauma responses that are part of the inheritance for our species' survival.

Mindfully revisiting these adaptive responses to trauma safely frees the response frozen in the tissues, allowing us to release the trauma burdens and return to a ventral vagal state. We start with noticing our movements that indicate which branch is dominant—the sympathetic branch (fight or flight), or the dorsal vagal part of the parasympathetic branch (freeze, appease)—so that we can find the traumatized Parts and help the ANS shift towards the ventral vagal state of social engagement. Trembling, shaking, and twitching indicate the trauma held in the tissues is releasing.

SAFETY GUIDELINES

Track your sensations, breath, heart, and gut to gauge your level of activation. Use any tools you learned in the last three chapters to return safety and calm to your inner system.

Feel free to pause or to skip any exercise.

EXPERIENTIAL EXERCISE
MOVEMENT AND OUR ANS—SYMPATHETIC ACTIVATION

1. Recall a challenging situation that you perceived could be threatening, and so you felt compelled to get away, or where you were preparing to have to defend yourself. Choose a memory that is not too activating or upsetting—perhaps one that you have worked with but not yet explored through movement.

2. What images, thoughts, and feelings arise?

3. As you stay with this memory, what do you notice about your heart rate?

4. What movements or movement impulses do you notice in your eyes, arms, and legs?

5. How do you feel towards these movements?

6. Remembering these movements are inherited and adaptive to our survival, let the movements know they are appreciated.

7. Mindfully explore these movements, welcoming their expression, frequently pausing to notice your internal state and to rest.

EXPERIENTIAL EXERCISE
MOVEMENT AND OUR ANS—PARASYMPATHETIC (DORSAL VAGAL)

1. Recall a challenging situation where you felt stuck, trapped, withdrawn, unable to escape. You just had to endure it, and you did so by spacing out or shutting down. Again, choose a situation that is only mildly activating.

2. What do you notice with your body (your posture, body awareness, energy level)?

3. Are there thoughts, words, emotions that arise?

4. Appreciate your Part for its intention to help you in this situation.

5. What does the Part need to hear from you?

6. Do you sense a movement that wants to happen but is blocked? What do you imagine would happen if you were to act on the impulse? Could you experiment with a small, slow, subtle, mindful expression of the movement?

7. If you find a place in your body that seems numb, outside your awareness, or immobilized, experiment with gently introducing movement. What happens? If your ANS shifts from this dorsal vagal state to a sympathetic state, you may feel an impulse to fight or flee. If your Parts agree, allow the impulse to be expressed while you mindfully witness the movement.

8. Take frequent pauses to rest and attend to your internal bodymind system.

EXPERIENTIAL EXERCISE
MOVEMENT AND OUR ANS—APPEASE

1. Recall a challenging situation involving a person who was in a position of power where you felt a lack of safety. Instead of trying to get away or shut down, your instinctual people-pleasing strategy to survive kicked in.

2. What Parts of you were exiled?

3. What words describe how you felt?

4. What happens in your body?

5. How did this strategy serve you?

6. Pause. Shake off the energy and movements of appeasement.

7. Thank your Part. Acknowledge how it helped you. Ask when it first learned this strategy.

8. Ask this Part what it needs to trust You with similar situations in the future.

EXPERIENTIAL EXERCISE
MOVEMENT AND OUR ANS—PARASYMPATHETIC (VENTRAL VAGAL)

1. Recall a challenging situation where you succeeded in navigating the challenge.

2. What supported you to meet the challenge?

3. What do you feel in your body?

4. Imagine sharing this success with a person or people you feel safe with.

5. Notice your movement impulses (rest, relax, smile, breathe, celebrate) and give them expression.

EXPERIENTIAL EXERCISE
MOVEMENTS TO RETURN THE ANS TO THE VENTRAL VAGAL STATE

1. Any movement done mindfully.

2. Aerobic exercises (avoid overtraining).

3. Dancing, especially with others.

4. Playing a musical instrument.

5. Humming, singing, chanting, gargling.

6. Deep, slow, diaphragmatic breathing.

7. Crossing your arms; pat your shoulders or upper arms.

8. Cross-lateral movements with arms and legs.

9. Lying on your back, interweave your fingers and place them behind your head; look to the right without turning your head; remain until you spontaneously yawn or swallow. Return your eyes to the neutral state; repeat on the left side.

10. Placing your tongue in front of your teeth, move your tongue clockwise towards the right cheek, the lower teeth, the left cheek, and back to the front teeth. Move your tongue counterclockwise. Experiment with the pace and length of time.

11. Exposure to cold: a cold shower, a dip in a frigid body of water, dunk your face in cold water.

Mindful Movement with Front and Back Body

In addition to connecting with the earth and sky through our body awareness (refer to chapters 2 and 3), we draw from the different qualities of our front body and back body as we move. Our front bodies are soft; our back bodies are strong. Our front and back bodies also have developed in different ways when we were embryos. Just days after conception, cells begin to organize themselves into two flat pancakes. One became the front body, known as the endoderm; the other became the back body, known as the ectoderm. These two bodies have two different functions. Out of the front body emerged a yolk sac, which later became the digestive organs. Out of the back body emerged the protective amniotic sac, which morphed into the nervous system and skin. Our front body and back body have been assisting our needs for nourishment and protection since before our birth. Today they offer different qualities to our movement.

EXPERIENTIAL EXERCISE
FRONT AND BACK BODY IN RELATIONSHIP AND MOVEMENT
Front Body

1. Lying on your back or sitting on the floor in a comfortable position, tune in to your front body. Touch it from your head to your toes. Feel the softness, openness, juiciness from your mouth all the way down past your gut to your anus.

2. Bring your hand to your navel where you first received nourishment. Breathe in and out through your navel.

3. Lie on your stomach, maybe with a bolster underneath your belly. Take time for your front body to meet the earth. Feel all the places that make contact with the floor. Bring your breath to your entire front body. What do you notice (vibrations, emotions, images, sensations, impulses)?

4. What are some of the qualities of your front body?

5. Do you find any Parts?

6. Begin to move from your front body—slithering, crawling, flexing the front body. Eventually come to an upright standing posture. Take a few steps forward, leading with your mouth, then your navel, then your gut, then your entire front body. What can your front body receive from the outside world?

7. What do you notice (vibrations, emotions, images, sensations, impulses)?

8. Do you find any Parts?

9. Imagine a person is in front of you. Move towards that person from your front body. What do you notice (vibrations, emotions, images, sensations, impulses)?

10. Do you find any Parts?

Back Body

1. Lie on your back with a blanket under your body. Tune in to your back body, noticing all the places your body makes contact with the floor. Yield into the earth. Bring your breath to your entire back body. Pull the blanket around you to replicate the origins of this ectoderm—the amniotic sac that provides a protective bubble that encases the developing front body.

2. What do you notice (vibrations, emotions, images, sensations, impulses)?

3. As your back body eventually became your skin and nervous system, touch your skin where you can reach from the back of your head to your heels. What are some of the qualities of your back body?

4. Do you find any Parts connected with your back body?

5. Begin to move from your back body, flexing and extending your back body. Let your back body guide you to come to standing. Take a few steps, moving from your back body. How does your back body serve you as you step out into the world?

6. Imagine a person is in front of you. Move towards that person from your back body. What do you notice (vibrations, emotions, images, sensations, impulses)?

7. Do you find any Parts?

Front and Back Body

1. Play with moving towards different people, from your front body and then your back body.

2. What have you learned about the qualities of your front body and back body that can help you maintain or bring Self energy to relationships?

Restoring the Flow with the Five Movements:
Yield, Push, Reach, Grasp, Pull

We revisit our earliest movements from conception to infancy because they are the basis for our later development. Not just our motor development, but also our physical, social, cognitive, and emotional development. As adults, we may have difficulty with letting go, reaching out, pushing away, holding on, or moving forward in life. We may have resistance or aversions to moving, or to some kind of movements with some parts of our bodies. Although we have worked with Parts connected with these difficulties, if we have not yet found a resolution, we may need to dig deeper and earlier.

Although the events or situations that led to our earliest burdens may be far outside our conscious awareness, they can be accessed with Mindful Movement. We can find these Parts that have been waiting all these many years to be seen, heard, witnessed, and resonated with in order to be freed of their burdens that, although lost to conscious memory, are held in implicit memory in our tissues and continue to influence many aspects of our lives. We find these very young Parts for whom movement was the primary means to sense, connect, communicate, and explore themselves and their relationship to their world.

We enter the preverbal matrix of our embryological and early infant movement experiences by mindfully revisiting each of five basic movements as they sequence through our bodies. We somatically witness disruptions in the natural motor development from attachment trauma that have become locked in the muscles, bones, and nervous system. Intergenerational burdens can be accessed by revisiting these early movement patterns. Embryonic Parts may sense into the burdens of the mother or past generations.

Through movement we retrieve these Parts from their obscurity. We physically feel and resonate with how the desires, needs, and expressions of these young Parts were thwarted. We continue to explore the movement, and the sequence of movements, until the ease, flow, and grace of the movement is restored, indicating that the burdens are released and the early movements have been repatterned. The ripples flow through the fluidity of time and space to affect other areas where our natural early development was impeded.

We move throughout our lives, beginning with conception. Again, any delay or disruption in our natural unfolding may affect later movement patterns as well as our cognitive and emotional development. Mindful Movement is a way to access and witness these implicitly held memories. We consider the five sequential and interrelated movements that begin in the uterus and become the prototypes of our later physical and emotional development—yield, push, reach, grasp, and pull.

We bring mindful attention to the five sequential movements of yield, push, reach, grasp, and pull through our six limbs—head, tail, legs, and arms. The navel is at the center, the core of these movements. These movements express the reality of our unified wholeness, with differentiated yet connected Parts. Some of these movements may reawaken the delight and power of exploring and moving, first swimming in amniotic fluids, and then navigating the earthly world. We may find movements that feel unfamiliar, weak, disconnected, awkward, constrained, or even impossible. Some movements may feel easy and flowing with one part of our body, and sticky or jerky with another. Along with our open, sustained attention to our physical experience, we notice emotions, images, and memories that arise as they often add to the story of these very young Parts. Protector Parts also often arise, with dissociation or distraction. Other sensations may be felt, like nausea or a rapid heartbeat.

With this next exercise, we revisit and reenact these basic movements to discover any disturbances in motor development and to allow the frozen impulses and the associated emotions to sequence through the body, restoring our embryological wisdom, creativity, collaboration, and resilience. Burdens inherited or energetically transmitted intergenerationally can also be cleared in this way. We begin with revisiting, with our imagination and our bodies, the embryological movements that are the building blocks of locomotion and our earliest connection experiences.

Throughout this exercise, frequently pause and return to *yield* as home base to bring mindfulness to Parts' expressions in response to the movement. Record what you notice. Be open to thoughts, memories, emotions, images, and other sensations. You may choose to do these exercises with a partner or therapist.

EXPERIENTIAL EXERCISE
REVISITING EMBRYOLOGICAL MOTOR DEVELOPMENT

1. Lie down in a warm, comfortable place in a position that supports you. Imagine that you are a single fertilized cell floating in the amniotic waters—perhaps on your side in a fetal position.

2. Your skin is your cell membrane, breathing in and out. You rest deeply, surrendering, floating, pulsating with creativity. Feel the exchange of inner and outer fluid as you experience this first foundational movement—**yield.**

3. Allow enough time to experience this movement of yield. Yielding is the opposite of collapsing. You are present to your sensations, sensing your relationship with the earth, and allowing the ground to fully support you. Notice any muscles from head to toe that are tense and invite them to let go.

4. As you become a multicellular being, your cells communicate and collaborate and form your front and back body that you experienced in the earlier exercise. Place your hand on your navel as you imagine a stalk growing and reaching towards the uterine wall or towards the center of the earth. Imagine you are breathing in and out through this firmly attached umbilicus, with every cell receiving all that you need. Imagine freely floating while securely attached to this nourishment from your navel and protected by your back body. What do you notice: sensations, images, emotions?

5. Lie on your front body and experience yield in this position, continuing to breathe in and out through your navel. When your body has enjoyed enough of the movement of **yield,** you might feel the impulse to **push.** You can play with the movements of **yield** and **push** while lying on your front body. You might also want to experience these movements while lying on your back body. Pause to notice the different qualities of these two movements and how they relate to each other.

6. As you are securely attached through your navel to the womb receiving all you need, your body begins to grow structures that become your arms and legs. You can now

move from your six limbs—your head, tail, arms, and legs. Your six limbs easily glide through your watery world.

7. Play with the sequence of **yield** and **push** with each of your six limbs. Letting the push originate from the navel, push down with both arms, then each arm one at a time. Press with hands, then a finger. Push down with both legs together, then one at a time. Press with a foot, then a toe. Try light pressure, harder pressure. Return to yield to rest and reflect. Do you notice any differences as you experience these movements in your six limbs?

8. Open to any images, thoughts, or emotions that arise. What opportunities do yield and push provide you?

9. These movements prepare you to make the wondrous journey from your watery world to emerging onto solid land. But before we leave the womb, experiment with the movement **reach,** which you need to develop to prepare you for birth. Do the movements of yield and push support your **reach?** Try this movement through each of your limbs. What is the quality of this movement of reach? What do you notice as you compare reaching from each limb? What do you imagine you are reaching for?

10. Play with the sequential movements of **yield, push, reach,** and then pause for rest and reflection in **yield** to integrate your experiences.

11. Did any movements (**yield, push,** or **reach**) feel unfamiliar or uncomfortable? Through which limbs? Any associated emotions, images, or memories? Are there any movements that seem to want more attention? If so, mindfully explore the movement until you find a release leading to greater flow and ease. Welcome and witness any Parts that show up.

12. Did you uncover any burdened Parts from these movements? From your own earliest beginnings or from ancestral or intergenerational burdens? Did you experience an unburdening as you imagined or reenacted your earliest movement repertoire? Were any of the lost qualities restored?

EXPERIENTIAL EXERCISE

MOVING ON LAND; ONTOGENY AND PHYLOGENY

Having practiced these movements in the womb, they serve us on the journey to be born. The movement **reach** leads to **grasp** and **pull**—extending with the movement of reach and flexing with the movements of grasp and pull. Our motor development in some ways parallels the development of the evolution of our species, from single-celled organisms to mammals. A playful way to explore and repattern our own early motor development experiences is through enacting the movement of these creatures. In the womb, we reimagined being a one-celled organism. As cells multiply, we become a sponge. Then we can play a six-limbed starfish, receiving our nourishment through our navel and using push and reach to move through the ocean. With our vertical alignment, we can resonate with the movements of primitive vertebrate animals like snakes and fish.

1. Let's begin with playing starfish. Lie on your stomach and imagine you are lying on a rock in the ocean, receiving nourishment through your center. Push and reach with each of your limbs from your center.

2. Still lying on your stomach, become a snake. Feel the length of your spine. Sliver, slide, and wiggle along the floor, using yield, push, and reach to move. Reach with your sense organs of your head—your eyes, mouth, ears, and nose—for nourishment and safety.

3. Play with yield, push, and reach to roll onto your side and your back. What animal do you feel like?

4. Play frog. Yield on your lily pad and push to sitting. You are hungry. You see a dragonfly. You push from your tail and both back legs, and reach with both front legs and your head. You grasp your dinner and pull it towards your mouth. Return to yield to digest your meal.

5. Play lizard, again lying on your stomach. Extend and reach with your limbs on your left side while you flex and push with your limbs on your right side. Continue with these homolateral movements as you move across the floor.

6. Become a mammal. Come to all fours. Reach with your right arm as you push with your left leg. Your right arm yields and pushes as the left leg reaches. Continue with these diagonal, contralateral movements. Play with other ways of moving, using yield, push, and reach with your six limbs.

7. When you find an object you want, move towards that, and when you reach it, grasp it and pull it towards you.

8. Play a primate: if you feel an impulse to stand or walk, you are not only playing monkey or chimp, you are completing the stages of movements from conception to the first year of life. Use the five movements to come to standing and take a few steps.

9. Return to yield to rest and reflect.

EXPERIENTIAL EXERCISE
REFLECTION ON THE FIVE MOVEMENTS

1. Which of these following aspects of each of the movements did you experience?

   ❏ Yield: Oneness. Relationship to earth. Surrender. Letting go. State of being. Effortlessly receive nourishment.

❏ Push: Differentiate. Assert separateness while connected. Relationship to surrounding space. Right to boundary. Verticality.

❏ Reach: Affirm desires and needs. Express desires and needs.

❏ Grasp: Connect, claim, hold on.

❏ Pull: Completion of the previous movements.

2. Are there other ways you would describe the meaning, opportunity, or quality of each of the five movements as you experienced them?

3. Which of the five movements were a challenge for you? Through which of your six limbs?

4. What emotions, sensations, memories, or images came up?

5. Did you imagine what you were pushing away, reaching for, grasping, or pulling towards you?

6. What Parts came up as you explored the movements? Do you have a sense of the Parts' story?

7. Did you have an experience of restoring the ease and flow of a movement that was challenging at first?

8. Is there a movement that was too challenging to do at this time?

9. Are there movements you want to revisit?

10. Consider one of your everyday movements in terms of these five movements and your six limbs: dancing, yoga, fitness exercises, gardening, housework, sports.

Using Mindful Movement Exercises with a Partner or a Group

Any one of the previous exercises could be enhanced by doing it with a partner, and possibly switching roles. Being with even one person is an antidote to our social isolation, expressing the truth of our interdependence and the benefits of coregulation as we dive deeply to explore the pain and wisdom held in our bodies as expressed through movement. Many of the exercises can be adapted to be used in a group setting. The transformations that happen in our Somatic IFS programs have demonstrated the exponential power of collective healing.

1. Your partner reads the instructions and listens to your reflection and sharing after the exercise.

2. Your partner mirrors your habitual movement pattern while you witness your Part as it is externalized.

3. You reach towards your partner, or push against them with your six limbs.

4. Your partner holds resonant Self energy to witness your Part's movement story.

5. Both sing, hum, and dance together to restore the ventral vagal state.

Mindful Movement to Heal Ancestral Burdens

We have explored movements of Parts and Self in our internal systems, movements associated with unresolved trauma, and movements from our earliest experiences in the womb and infancy. Some of our habitual movements may not be related to our own individual life experiences. The source of some of our movements may be intergenerational or ancestral. Our everyday, largely unconscious movements may have originated in traumatic experiences of our parents, grandparents, or even ancient ancestors through bodily inheritance and culturally defining experiences (refer to chapter 4). Just as our movements can reveal the implicitly held memories of our earliest experiences, they can lead us to our legacy burdens, allowing a release of the burden stored in our cells, nervous systems, and muscles and fascia, and ending the cycle of unprocessed trauma carried through the generations.

Mindful Movement for Social Transformation

Movement can be a path not only for our individual liberation from our traumas, but also towards healing societal burdens. Individually, we can feel isolated and powerless as we experience societal burdens. Collectively, we identify movements of our burdened Parts associated with our social identities.

NOTE

Recall the preceding chapter on "Radical Resonance" and the section titled "Embodied Social Identity."

You named some of your social identities—some are valued and assigned power and privilege, while others are devalued by our culture.

Individually and collectively, our bodies are shaped by social systems that define our identities that deeply affect our lives. Our social identities affect how we move through the world to meet our survival needs for safety, belonging, and dignity. Depending on whether our identities are valued by society or not, we tighten up or go slack, we move towards or away, we puff up or shrink, we look to fight or appease. For survival, individually and collectively, we mimic what is valued and exile or reject what is devalued.

Whether we identify as a member of a dominant group or an oppressed or marginalized group, our movements are determined by burdened Parts and do not flow freely. Because we have embodied and have been shaped by systems built on exercising power over others and nature, we need to transform these experiences and develop collective practices that grow from a premise of interdependence. You might want to consider first doing this exercise on your own, and then bringing it to a group, either a group with similar or different social identities. You can embody and move any of the social identities you are curious about regardless of whether it is an identity that you claim.

EXPERIENTIAL EXERCISE
EMBODYING OUR SOCIAL IDENTITIES THROUGH MOVEMENT

1. Focus on one of your privileged identities. Consider how you and others with that identity have embodied the belief that your *perceived* safety, belonging, and dignity are based on domination and the centering of that privileged identity, assuming that it is the defining norm.

2. Embody this belief or attitude of supremacy and privilege. Let it move you through space. Exaggerate it. How does your body express this in your posture, gait, gestures?

3. Do you find Parts that need to feel superior to feel OK? If so, ask these Parts if they are from your life or if they are inherited from an ancestor. How does movement help you understand these Parts? If there is discomfort, try to stay with it and let the discomfort move you.

4. Play with expressing each of the five movements from the perspective of this identity. What are your Parts reaching for? Pushing away? Grasping?

5. What would your Parts need to be able to let go of the movements, and the burdened beliefs and emotions, associated with dominance and privilege that they have adopted? From the wisdom and creativity of Embodied Self, how might you use the privileges of your dominant social identities?

6. Choose one of the identities not valued by society, either one of your identities or one that you want to explore. Embody this identity and express it in movements.

7. What burdens do you carry from societal oppression of your identity? How do these survival strategies meet your internal system's need for safety, belonging, or dignity? When and how do they serve you, and how not? Are there movements that express the burdens and survival strategies?

8. Imagine that you live in a world where all bodily differences are equally valued. Move in that world. What is different in your movements? In your emotions, thoughts, and energy?

9. How might Mindful Movement be a path to societal transformation?

Clinical Application of Mindful Movement
Bringing Mindful Movement into the Session

We begin with ourselves as therapists to mindfully explore our relationship to movement. Most of us, unless we are specialists in dance and movement, expect that we and our clients will remain seated throughout the session. We do not pay much attention to our clients' spontaneous movements or blocked movement impulses that may be signaling a message from a Part. We typically do not consider suggesting movements to our clients at any stage of the therapeutic process. Our internal systems may carry burdens regarding our movement histories. We may fear triggering our client's resistance to move. Our Parts and our Self energy are conveyed through our gestures, posture, and stance implicitly transmitting our emotions and energies to our clients.

1. What is your experience with using movement in therapy, either as a client or as a therapist?

   _____

   _____

   _____

2. If you typically do not use movement, what concerns come up as you imagine integrating movement into your practice?

   _____

   _____

   _____

3. What movement practices help you cultivate and sustain your Embodied Self energy?

   _____

   _____

   _____

4. Are there any brief movements you use in between sessions to restore your Self energy?

   _____

   _____

   _____

EXPERIENTIAL EXERCISE
MINDFUL MOVEMENTS FOR THE THERAPIST

1. As you begin a session, relax your muscles around your eyes, jaw, and mouth. Lengthen the back of your neck. Drop your shoulder blades and your sacrum.

2. Make any other changes in your posture that will allow you to feel connected with above and below, and allow free and full breaths.

3. Use some gentle movements for any other muscle tension or lack of muscle tone.

4. Consider movements to restore Embodied Self energy during those few minutes between client sessions.

5. Gently tap up and down along the sternocleidomastoid muscle of your neck to shift your ANS to the ventral vagal state.

6. Track your own movements or movement impulses during the session, moving towards or away from the client for indications of Parts—your own Parts or Parts in the relational field.

7. Notice whether you unconsciously mirror your clients' movements during a session.

As with the other Somatic IFS practices, Mindful Movement can facilitate all the steps of the IFS process, from accessing a Part that may only be found in movement to integrating the transformations. Opportunities for bringing this practice into the session flow naturally from the other Somatic IFS practices. The practice of Somatic Awareness may find a sensation that leads to a Part's movement story that wants to unfold, sequence, and be witnessed. Breathing involves movement, and moving depends on and assists breathing. A resonant therapist may consciously or unconsciously mirror the client's movements or feel movement impulses in their own body that the client's Parts have disallowed. The Somatic IFS therapist, attending to the client's nonverbal right-brain expressions, relies on their resonant capacity to sense when to invite their client to bring their awareness to their movement and when to suggest movements to facilitate the therapeutic process.

SOME SUGGESTIONS TO HELP BRING MINDFUL MOVEMENT INTO YOUR THERAPEUTIC SESSIONS

- When a Part shows up initially as an emotion or thought: "As you stay with this emotion or thought, is there a movement that can express this?"

- When a client is reporting, narrating, and explaining their situation and you sense their protector Parts may be avoiding going deeper: "Let's take a pause with the story to see if there is a movement that can express what you have been talking about." "I am noticing your leg is jiggling as you talk. Let's take a moment to stay with that jiggling to see what it might be wanting us to know."

- Track for any movements in any part of the body during the session with the same attention you give to the client's verbal communication. Consider when and if to invite the client's awareness of these spontaneous, largely unconscious movements: "I am noticing your hands are gripping the chair as you speak of this. Would it be OK to pause the story to bring your full attention to your hands to see what this movement may be adding to your story?"

- When the client speaks in words that indicate movement, like feeling stuck, trapped, torn, wanting to get away, hold on, or back off: "Can you find a movement that expresses this feeling?"

- To get to know a protector Part: "Let's ask this Part to show us how it behaves in your system to keep things under control." "Your body just got rigid as you began to share that with me. Could that be coming from a Part that is concerned?" "Can the Part show you what it is afraid would happen?" "Can this Part show you how it protects you?"

- When Parts are polarized: "Would each of these Parts be willing to show you and me how they feel towards the other Part?"

- The stories of the vulnerable, exiled Parts can be witnessed through movement: "I am noticing your body curling inward/collapsing/getting agitated. Stay with this movement and see where it takes you." "Do you want to show how trapped your Part felt?" "I can see your arms are beginning to tremble. That is a good sign. The trauma stored in your body is releasing. Let it happen; let it get as big as it wants to be."

- Providing an opportunity to experience the missing, disallowed experience: "If you could get away from this scary situation, how would you do that?" "It was too scary to push him away back then. Do you want to try it with me right now?" "There was no one there when you tried to reach out. Would you like to reach out towards me right now?" "There was no way to escape. If it had been possible, how would you have gotten free?" "Are you ready to leave this place you've been hiding? Do you want to walk, run, or crawl? Shall I do it with you?" "Ahh, you are now able to relax. Let that happen even more. Enjoy that."

- Suggesting movements for unburdening: "Now that your Parts are ready to let go of this burden, how would they like to do that? Do you want to throw, kick, bury, or burn the burden? Do you want to trample on it, tear it up, or smash it?"

- Restoring the lost qualities: "Is there a movement that can express this feeling of openness/freedom/relief/safety/innocence?" "Can you imagine this little one playing/resting?"

- Integration: "Is there a movement that can express this new courage and confidence?" "Would the Part like you to repeat and practice this movement to help remind this Part of what is possible?" "Is there a movement that can help this Part hold on to the change?"

Integration of Mindful Movement

We have explored and experienced our habitual gestures, postures, and gaits, our early developmental movements, and movements that have been inhibited or suppressed. Bringing mindful awareness to these movements or lack of movements, we have accessed both Parts and Self of our bodymind systems. Movement, as the primal language of our emotions, is a gateway to our Parts. When our Parts' implicit stories can be known, witnessed, and unburdened through the practice of Mindful Movement, we have found a path to greater Embodied Self energy. The following exercises can integrate and anchor the expression of Embodied Self through movement. Then we bring this energy to our final practice in the next chapter, "Attuned Touch."

EXPERIENTIAL EXERCISE
MOVEMENTS TO CULTIVATE EMBODIED SELF

1. Do you have movement practices that express and support your true nature, that bring out who you truly are at your best?

2. What movements do you most enjoy?

3. Each of the movements in the next exercise can connect you with your Self energy. As you try each of them, consider the following questions:

- Which works best for you?
- Which do you enjoy the most?
- Which could be helpful when your Parts take over?
- Which might you want to include in a daily practice?

EXPERIENTIAL EXERCISE
MOVEMENTS TO EXPRESS EMBODIED SELF

1. Connecting with heaven and earth

- Standing, reach towards the earth with one arm, and reach towards the sky with the other arm, enjoying the length of the stretch.
- Alternate reaching downwards with one arm and upwards with the other arm.
- Bring your arms and hands to join at your heart.
- Continue with these movements, coordinating them with your breathing.

2. Tuning in to your natural rhythms

- Find a quiet, private place to sit or lie down comfortably.
- Notice the movements in your body that are happening even in stillness—heartbeat, breathing, fluids flowing in your digestive organs, the subtle long waves produced by cerebrospinal fluid, the pulsations and vibrations in your cells.
- Choose one of these movements to focus on for several minutes.

3. The 8 C's of Self energy

- Remember, the qualities that describe Self energy include compassion, clarity, courage, connection, calmness, confidence, curiosity, and creativity.

- Move from each of these qualities. Include posture, gestures, facial expressions, and gait.

- Include the five movements with all six limbs.

- Experiment with the pace of the movement and the intensity of the expression.

4. Free-form movements

- Play music; let the music move your body.

- Outside in nature, notice all that is moving—trees, leaves, grass, clouds, insects, birds, squirrels. Focus on one of the movements. Let your body join the movement dance.

- Letting go of movements you have studied or learned, give your body permission to move you in any way.

6

Attuned Touch

Purpose of Attuned Touch

THIS FINAL PRACTICE of Attuned Touch, held and embraced by each of the four interdependent practices that precede it, is the jewel on the crown of the Somatic IFS practices. Resting at the top of the Somatic IFS Logo, Attuned Touch returns us to the roots of our implicit communication between Parts and Self. Somatic IFS welcomes this practice from its place of exile, where, because of its association with sexuality, power, and abuse, it has lain hidden in the shadows of fear and shame. Attuned Touch, whether it is imaginary touch, self touch, or touch from another person, can heal the wounds from touch neglect and abuse, restoring our birthright of sensory aliveness and linking Somatic IFS with healing and spiritual practices throughout the ages.

Touch has been used for healing and bonding by humans and many other animals. More recently, the use of touch for healing has been controversial in the psychotherapy community. The potential of touch for healing bodies, minds, and cultures, and the equal potential of touch to do harm, calls for safeguards to ensure that this overlooked communication pathway is used judiciously, wisely, ethically, appropriately, effectively, and with permission of all the Parts. To harness the healing potential of this intervention while avoiding harmful touch, the Somatic IFS therapist relies on the practices of awareness, breathing, resonance, and movement. Attuned Touch also draws on all four of the elements associated with the Somatic IFS practices—earth, air, water, and fire—to guide our touch.

Consider how touch is our first language. It is connected at the most primitive level with protection and communication, beginning within days after conception. The embryo's protective amniotic sac morphs into the tactile system. The fetus develops these systems through movement as it floats in its primeval sea and begins to know itself as it bounces against the uterine wall. The connection between our nervous and tactile systems continues as our bodies develop, serving both communication and protection. Our nervous systems have pathways to and from the brain and the skin. Receptors in our brains receive and encode sensory information about touch and make meaning of it. Throughout our lives, touch remains a powerful channel of implicit, nonverbal communication.

> After birth, touch continues to be the primary language of the infant. The warm, sensual, physical contact between infant and caregiver establishes a bonding even more crucial than food for healthy development. Touch is a building block of secure attachment. When the touch is attuned to the infant, communicating security, safety, and belonging, the infant develops the secure attachment that becomes the foundation for their later relational lives. Not enough touch, or the wrong kind of touch, results in developmental trauma and lifelong adverse ramifications. For Parts with wounds of attachment, as with our clients' infant or pre-birth Parts, touch can be the most effective communication. Tactile experiences remain central to our emotions, our thought processes, and our healing throughout our life.[1]

When touch is attuned, appropriate, safe, and respectful of all Parts in the system, these positive sensory experiences create new neural patterns and release oxytocin, a hormone that solidifies a trusting bond between the Part and Self. Attuned Touch in Somatic IFS includes exercises involving all three kinds of touch: imaginary touch, our self touch, and touch from another person, including the therapist.

Depending on your personal touch history and culture, your inner system will be your guide as you consider the exercises in this chapter. In some cases, self touch or imaginary touch may pave the way to receive touch from another person. We will begin with exploring your history of touch. As you read and respond to the following questions, your body will let you know when your Parts are activated by the memory. You can decide when to take a pause, skip the question, or ask a friend or therapist to be present with you.

Individual Application of Attuned Touch
Elements

As mentioned, the classical elements of earth, air, water, and fire that have been used to explain physical bodies as well as metaphysical phenomena have also been associated with the first four of the Somatic IFS practices. This fifth practice, just as it relies on the four prior practices to support our touch, unites these four elements. My bodywork teachers emphasized the importance of grounding before making physical contact with an earthy, fleshy body. A few deep in-breaths bring spaciousness, and Parts with agendas or concerns can let go on the out-breath. We feel the rhythms and waves of the tissue under our hands and restore fluidity to frozen and numb places. The transformative aspect of fire is conveyed in a warm hand fueled by a compassionate heart. All these elements link the Somatic IFS practices with healing and spiritual practices throughout the ages.

Personal Touch History

Awareness of our touch histories is crucial for the practice of ethical Attuned Touch. Below are some questions to help you consider your experiences of touch throughout your life. If you experience Parts being activated during this, the Somatic IFS practices can be a resource to bring Embodied Self to the burdened Parts.

Before the questions, we will start with recalling a memory of safe, loving, healing, welcome touch. Stay with the memory, including all the senses and bodily experiences connected with this touch. This memory can be a "touch stone" if any of the following questions activate your Parts.

1. What is your earliest touch memory?

   _____

   _____

   _____

2. Did your experience of being touched, or not being touched, change during your childhood and adolescence? Include significant memories of touch from medical professionals, sports, friends.

   _____

   _____

   _____

3. What do you remember of touch experiences in your early adulthood?

   _____

   _____

   _____

4. What role did your family, race, religion, or other cultural factors play in your touch history?

   _____

   _____

   _____

5. To what degree does your history of touch influence your touch experiences today, personally and professionally?

   _____

   _____

   _____

NOTE

You may want to journal, draw and name Parts, or create a timeline.

---

6. Did you find a Part that did not receive enough touch? A Part that received unwelcome touch, or not the right kind of touch? Can the 6 F's help you with this Part? Would this Part be open to receiving touch from You?

_____

_____

_____

The burdens from touch can affect the ability of our tactile systems to accurately receive information from our environment, causing hyper- or hyposensitivity. Receptors on our skin, nerves, and muscles send information to the brain, which interprets and responds to the information. The upcoming exercise brings awareness to this sensory process, which is fundamental to our well-being and all our interactions with the world.

Imaginary Touch

Imaginary Attuned Touch is commonly seen in an IFS session when a Part, often an exile, spontaneously leaps into the client's lap, leans into them, or clings to them. Staying with this movement deepens the relationship between Self and the vulnerable Part and secures the Part's new experience of safe connection.

Imaginary touch may be used with Parts not yet ready for direct physical contact. As we imagine holding a Part of ourselves, or that Part being held by someone safe, we experience many of the benefits of actual physical contact from ourselves or another. With Parts that have wounds from touch neglect, we can imagine those Parts being held, caressed, and hugged. With Parts with wounds from touch abuse or who have an aversion to touch, we imagine appropriate, safe touch from a person who respects boundaries as well as being able to say no to unwanted touch. Even imaginary touch releases the hormone oxytocin to foster a safe, resonant Self-to-Part relationship. Imaginary touch can:

- Affect physiology—blood pressure, heart rate, hormones, immune system
- Help with distorted body image
- Assist with awareness and appreciation of the body
- Calm the ANS
- Restore healthy boundaries
- Awaken your tactile system

EXPERIENTIAL EXERCISE
AWAKENING YOUR TACTILE SYSTEM

1. Your skin is your largest organ, covering, containing, and protecting your entire body. Bring your awareness to your entire skin.

2. How do you feel towards your skin?

3. Touch the skin of a part of your body with an object. Touch the skin of a part of your body with your hand. How do these different touches affect your degree of sensitivity for this part of your body? How do they affect how you feel towards this part of your body?

4. Explore the textures of objects near you with different parts of your body. What parts of your body are most sensitive, least sensitive? What happens to these parts of your body as you touch different objects? How does touch affect your degree of sensitivity?

5. Focus on the skin and muscles of your hand. Awaken the senses in your hand by touching an object. Compare the sensations as you touch with your palm, fingers, and the back of your hand.

6. Invite a Part to do the touching of an object. You might want to invite a vulnerable Part that needs touch or that fears it, a firefighter Part that uses touch to soothe or distract, or a manager Part that uses touch to contain, control, or fix.

7. Focus on your heart. Direct energy from your heart through your arm to your hand. Touch an object or a part of your body with your hand.

8. Embody one of the qualities of Self energy. Touch from one of those qualities.

Self Touch

These exercises for self touch involve consciously sending Embodied Self energy to the place or Part in the body. They can be easily adapted to giving and receiving Attuned Touch with another person. Self touch in Somatic IFS also considers our habitual or spontaneous touch that we might want to explore more deeply to find a Part. Our touch might point to Parts in our body. Our hand might fly to our chest to bring protection, or to indicate that our speech is coming from a Part that resides there. We bring our awareness to our automatic touching. We slow it down, repeat the touch. We consider whether the touch is from Self or a Part, and whether the place being touched, or the Part doing the touching, is needing our Self-led self touch.

EXPERIENTIAL EXERCISE
ATTUNED SELF TOUCH

1. Find a place in your body that wants your touch.

    - Where in your body is this place?

    - What tells you this place wants touch? What sensations do you find here?

    - How do you feel towards this place?

    - Is this a place in your body needing touch, or is there a Part inhabiting this place in your body? Is it both, or unclear?

2. Prepare to touch in an attuned way.

    - Establish your inner vertical alignment. Ground with the earth; breathe in the Self energy around you. Focus on the hand that will be touching. Awaken the senses in your touching hand with awareness, touch, and movement.

    - How do you feel towards this place in your body that would like some touch?

    - Breathe into your heart to awaken your Self energy. Send this Self energy from your heart to your touching hand so it is open to giving and receiving.

    - Bring your awareness to the place in your body that wants touch from you. Let this place know it is in charge of the touch. Send a gentle inquiry to this place to let you know what kind of touch it would like.

3. Touching.

    - Slowly and mindfully move your hand towards this place. As your hand makes physical contact with this place in your body, use the movement of *yield* as your hand melts into a state of oneness with the skin and tissues below. You are communicating a state of "being with" to this place in your body.

    - Through your touch, transmit your Self energy to this place you are touching.

    - Listen with your hand to the responses to your touch—the skin, muscles, fascia, bones, blood, energy. What do you notice: sensations, thoughts, words, emotions, images?

    - You might sense this place is content with your touch, or perhaps it might want a different touch, or it might be open to experiencing a gentle *push,* a subtle *reach,* or a *grasp* and *pull* to contact the deeper levels of tissue and Parts that dwell there. Consider the pressure, movement, and duration that best sends your Self energy to this place in your body receiving the touch.

    - You can experiment with your touch, letting your body guide your touch, trusting this relationship between your hand conveying Self energy and this place in your body.

4. Completion.

- How do you sense when the touch is complete?

- What do you notice in your hand, in the place you were touching, and elsewhere in your body?

- Did you find a Part connected with the place you touched? If so, how is the Part now? Does this Part carry any touch burdens?

- Did any other Parts show up as you did this exercise?

EXPERIENTIAL EXERCISE
SELF-TO-PART COMMUNICATION THROUGH TOUCH

This exercise is a guide to bringing our Attuned Touch to a Part.

1. We begin with separating from any burdened Parts:

- Parts with touch techniques or protocols

- Parts that feel insecure because of lack of training or experience with touching

- Parts with agendas for the touch to result in a particular outcome

- Parts that carry wounds from touch

- Parts that polarize with the Part being touched

- Other Parts

2. Is there a Part you would like to connect with through touch? Where is this Part in your body?

3. Are there any other Parts concerned about this first Part receiving your touch?

4. Rub your palms together, breathe into your heart, and send your Self energy to your hand.

5. When your Part is ready for touch, make physical contact with this Part in your body as you did in the previous exercise.

6. Listen with your hand to this Part. Are there sensations or subtle movements or energies you feel? Do you notice emotions, images, thoughts, sensations, changes in your breathing, or movements elsewhere in your body?

7. You can communicate verbally, spoken aloud or silently, to the Part in your body, such as:

- "What would you like me to know about you?"

- "I am here. I'm listening. I hear you. It's OK now."

- "Is this touch just right, or would you like something different?"
- "What is my touch saying to you?"
- "What are you wanting me to know?"

8. When your Part feels complete with the touch, stay connected with the Part energetically as you gently remove your hand from this place in your body.

9. How is the Part after having received this touch from You?

With the next exercise, we start with a positive memory to provide a place to return to as you explore a Part with touch burdens. As you invite a Part that carries burdens from touch, choose a Part with what you consider a mild experience of not receiving the touch you wanted, a time you felt annoyed or disappointed. If a memory arises that is too painful for your system, ask it to not take over and then return to the first positive memory.

EXPERIENTIAL EXERCISE
ATTUNED TOUCH WITH PARTS WITH TOUCH BURDENS

1. Remember a time when you received touch from another person that was welcome, loving, connecting, and healing. You might recall a light touch or a full-bodied embrace. Let the memory develop with sights, sounds, smells, and sensations. What do you notice as you remember these experiences? You can return to this memory at any time during this exercise.

2. Recall a memory when you received the wrong kind of touch. If it is a memory of abusive or painful touch, or an overwhelming sense of touch neglect, ask that memory and the Parts that arise to wait until you have the support of a therapist.

3. Notice what happens in your body as you remember your experience. Notice any sensations, breath, or movement.

4. If Parts emerge—protector Parts and young, vulnerable exiles—you can make a list or a body map of these Parts.

5. Select a protector Part to focus on first. Notice how you feel towards this Part. If you feel Self energy, send it to this Part and notice how the Part responds.

6. Ask this protector Part if it is OK for you to continue.

7. If so, invite a Part to come forward that would like to experience getting the kind of touch it would have wanted from You.

8. Check with Parts in your system to find out if they are all OK with this.

9. Let your Part know it is in charge of the touch—what kind of touch, and the duration.

10. Awaken the senses in your hand. Feel your compassion for this Part. Send this Self energy from your heart to your hand. Ground; breathe.

11. When the Part is ready, ask it where it would like to feel touch from your hand.

12. Communicate with the Part—verbally and nonverbally—to find out what kind of touch it wants, what kind of touch it does not want.

13. Stay fluid with your touch as the Part changes or moves around in your body. You may listen through your hand to the flesh underneath it, to the muscles and fascia, the body story of the Part. You might feel a warmth, a softening, maybe even some trembling. Words may occur to you that go with the touch you are sending to this Part from your heart and through your arm to your hand. See if the Part responds. Maybe there are other words the Part wants to hear. Let the words and feelings be expressed through your touch.

14. Ask the Part if it is ready to let go of a burden that went with this experience—a belief, feeling, or sensation. Maybe there is some further touch that can help with the unburdening process.

15. When your Part feels complete with the touch, stay connected with this Part energetically as you gently disconnect physically.

Restoring and Fostering Our Attuned Touch and Healthy Boundaries

We have a right to have our emotional and physical space respected. Many situations can occur during our lives in which we experience a violation of our space that leaves us feeling helpless and powerless. Very young people may be touched or held without their permission. Their needs for alone time, or connection with others, may not have been respected. More extreme violations include medical procedures, physical assault, combat, accidents, physical abuse or neglect, and sexual abuse. These situations result in a shattering of the integrity of a person's boundaries. Parts' burdens affect their ability to set healthy boundaries around touch. Attuned Touch can repair the ruptures, reinstating healthy boundaries.

EXPERIENTIAL EXERCISE
SAYING YES AND NO TO TOUCH

1. Find a time in your life, even recently, when you felt your emotional or physical space was not respected, or you were not able to state or defend your space. Choose a situation that will not be too activating.

2. What happened?

3. What Part or Parts arise with this memory? How do the Parts show up—emotions, images, sensations, thoughts?

4. How do you feel towards the Parts?

5. What burdens—sensations, emotions, behaviors, beliefs—have your Parts taken on as a result?

6. What difficulties do you experience in your current life from your Parts' burdens? Mark the ones that apply:

   ❑ Knowing when you do and don't want touch

   ❑ Knowing you have a right to say "yes" or "no" to touch

   ❑ Being able to say "yes" or "no" to touch

   ❑ Touching others with Self energy

   ❑ Receiving, appreciating, and enjoying touch from others

   ❑ Being able to distinguish safe, appropriate touch and unsafe touch

   ❑ Other:

   _____

   _____

   _____

7. Let your Parts know you understand and appreciate them, and that you can help them.

8. Ask your Parts:

   • Do you trust me to help you?

   • What do you wish had happened instead of what did happen?

   • Are you willing to imagine a scenario where this had happened?

   • Do you want to experience Self Touch with some part of your body?

   • How is it for you now? What has changed?

   • Which of your burdens can you let go of now?

Clinical Application of Attuned Touch

The cultural taboo against touch in psychotherapy encourages therapists to perpetuate the neglect that originally caused the injury. Because of the immense potential of touch to heal and to harm, this overlooked communication pathway . . . is

used judiciously and wisely in Somatic IFS, with permission of all the Parts. . . .
If it can be said that some psychotherapists are too cautious about touch, perhaps
bodyworkers and other health care professionals are not . . . sufficiently aware that
their touch may stir up trauma and other unresolved issues lying dormant in the
tissues of their clients' bodies.[2]

As a psychotherapist, having worked with your own touch burdens, aware of the risks and benefits
of touch, and supported by the previous Somatic IFS practices, you may be contemplating the
value of Attuned Touch with your clients. You may already be using touch in sessions with all of
your clients or with some of them. You might typically hug your clients, or some of your clients,
at the end of a session. Possibly you are considering what is being expressed or stirred up by those
hugs. Or you may have decided that touch between you and your clients is completely off the
table. If so, you have learned from this chapter about the value of imagined touch and the client's
self touch for addressing your client's physical and emotional issues. This section will address the
therapist's facilitation of imaginary touch with clients, the client's self touch, and finally, touch
from the therapist.

Touch, whether imaginary, self touch, or touch from a trusted professional, has been shown to be
beneficial in a wide range of clinical issues, such as anxiety, depression, hyperactivity, attention defi-
cits, grief, PTSD, and addictions. Studies have shown that the physiological and emotional effects of
trauma can be reversed through touch. Touch can repair wounds of attachment—emotionally, somatically, socially, even neurologically. Attuned Touch can bring physical healing as well, affecting every
system in the body, including cortisol levels, blood glucose, cardiac stress, immunity, pulmonary function, and blood pressure.

The proven power of touch for healing emotional and physical illness calls us to bring this practice
out of exile, "where it has lain hidden in the shadows of fear and shame because of its association with
sexuality, abuse, and violation."[3] Wounds of touch—touch neglect and touch abuse—are endemic in
many cultures, resulting in psychological and physiological burdens with life-long repercussions. For
example, research has revealed that babies in the United States receive less touch than in other nations,
and of the US babies, White babies receive the least touch. Other research on adult touch shows similar
results.

Touch finds Parts in the body as it awakens the dormant, usually wordless, and often imageless clues
to our psychological and cultural burdens where they are available for repair. Attuned Touch can keep
a focused attention on the Part. It can calm the nervous system, speaking directly to structures in the
brain to help the client unblend from dysregulated Parts. Touch can witness the Parts' stories as told
in the tissues as tightening, trembling, shaking, dissociating, softening, or melting. The client's inner
system receives a reparative experience as touch conveys an implicit message of safety and connection,
or comfort and pleasure. The young Parts securely attach with the client's Self, let go of past associations
of touch, and replace them with pleasurable experiences. In this way, the practice of Attuned Touch
restores our birthright of sensory aliveness and links Somatic IFS with healing and spiritual practices
throughout the ages.

Guiding the Client's Imaginary Touch

Many Somatic IFS therapists primarily use the client's self touch or imaginary touch with every step of the IFS Model. They or the client may prefer imaginary touch or the client's self touch instead of physical contact with the therapist. During the session, the client may report that they see or sense that a Part has engaged in touch.

The following are examples of what the therapist might say to support the imaginary touch happening in the client's internal system:

- "As you see, hear, or sense this Part, does it seem to want to be closer to you? Is that OK with you for it to do that?"

- "Ask the Part to get as close to you as it would like."

- "Would this Part that is holding on to you also like you to hold it?"

- "Is this touch just right for the Part?"

- "Stay with the Part as you are holding it. How does it seem, look, or feel to you now?"

- "Would this Part like to imagine the _____ is holding them like they always wanted?"

- "Would this Part like to tell this person to stop touching? Would this Part like you to hold their hand as they do this?"

- "Can this Part imagine being held by you for a short period of time? Maybe just their finger?"

Guiding the Client's Self Touch

The client's touch from their Embodied Self is in keeping with the essential premise of the IFS Model—that the Self of the client is the main agent of transformation. The client's Attuned Touch can foster a resonant relationship with their Part. The therapist can ask the client if this Part in their body would like touch. Touch can assist every step in the process of Somatic IFS therapy, from finding and focusing on the Part to witnessing and unburdening and to integration and completion.

As the Somatic IFS therapist is observing the nonverbal communication of their client, they may notice their client spontaneously touching a place on their body. Often a hand quickly lands on their chest when they experience a strong emotion. The client may habitually touch their forehead, cover their mouth, or scratch their head. The therapist can invite the client's awareness of this touch as it may be a Part's potent form of nonverbal communication. Together, regarding the largely unconscious touch with curiosity, they bring awareness to the grasping, scratching, rubbing, covering, holding, embracing, or slapping. They note the rate, pressure, intensity, duration, and incidence of the touch. The client is curious about who is doing the touching—is it their Self, or a Part?

The following are guidelines to explore the client's spontaneous touch:

- "I notice your hand has touched _____ several times. Are you interested to find out more about that?"

- "How are you feeling towards this place you are touching?"

- If it is a burdened Part doing the touching: "Are there words or emotions that are conveyed in the touch?" You might decide to shift your focus to this Part.

- If it is the client's Self energy doing the touching: "How is this touch for your Part? Is it just right, or would it prefer some different kind of touch? Would it like you to experiment with a different kind of touch—more pressure, a movement, a different place?"

- "What is your touch saying to this Part?" "What is the message the Part is getting from your hand?" "Would the Part like to hear those words?"

- "Are you getting any information from this Part/tissue you are touching? Can you let your Part know you are getting this?"

- "Let your Part know you will stay with it as long as it needs, and you will release your touch when it wants you to."

- "How is your Part now after having received the touch?"

- "Are there any other Parts that want to share how it was for them for your Part to receive your touch?"

The therapist can also direct the client's Self-led Attuned Touch to facilitate any step of the IFS Model with any Part.

- "I understand your protector Part hates this part of your body. At that time, this Part took on the belief that this part of your body was shameful/ugly/defective. How do You feel towards this part of your body?"

- "Would this place in your body be willing to experience through touch how You feel towards this part of your body?"

- "Maybe there is a kind of touch that can let this Part know you are here with it, that you want to get to know it better."

- "You tell me you are numb from the waist down. Would it be OK to bring your hand to the place just above your waist? What do you feel there? What is your hand saying to this place in your body? What do you notice with the numbness?"

- "This young Part you have found in your belly feels so alone and scared. Is there a touch that could help it feel safely connected with You? Would it like to try it? Are your other Parts OK with You touching this young Part in your belly? What is your touch saying to this young Part? What do you notice in your belly?"

- "Knowing it is in charge of the touch, is there a kind of touch that could bring safety, comfort, connection, or pleasure to your Part?"

- "We know this Part believes all touch is dangerous because of what happened when you were a child. Let this Part know we understand this, and we will not engage in touch unless and until this Part is OK with it."

- "Your Part is beginning to know and trust you. Is there a kind of touch that would help it even more to feel your presence, confidence, courage?"

- "I understand that another Part of you wants to receive some touch from you. Can you hold both of these Parts, one in each hand?"

The Therapist's Attuned Touch with the Client

Just as with the client's touch, the therapist needs to be in Embodied Self. Parts with an agenda to fix, correct, protect, or otherwise get our own needs met, Parts with fears or insecurities, are recognized and asked to move into the background to be worked with later as trailheads to our therapist Parts or our own touch histories.[4]

Although often the client's touch may be all their Part needs, in some cases safe touch from another trusted person can provide a needed experience to heal the wounds of touch. The therapist considers the client's relationship with their internal bodymind system, the state of the dyadic relational field, including the hierarchical and cultural aspects of their relationship, and the touch histories of both. If the therapist's Attuned Touch is appropriate, the therapist states the touch will not be sexual, that either of them can choose to stop the touch, and that the client is in charge of the touch.

The following are some verbal suggestions to facilitate the therapist's touch:

- "I see you are touching this place on your body. Is your touch alone just right, or would you like my touch instead, or in addition to your touch?"

- "You are letting me know you don't feel very grounded or connected. Do you think my touch could help? Perhaps my hands on the top of your feet?"

- "Are there any Parts that aren't sure they want this touch?"

- "Is there a kind of touch, or a place to touch, that might feel safe enough for a few seconds?"

- "I want you to know you are in charge of this touch. I want to get the touch just right for you. You can let me know when you want me to take away my hand, if you want more or less pressure, if the touch is just right."

- "Would you like to see if my physical connection with this place in your body might help you to keep your focus on it?"

- "What kind of touch did this young Part not get to experience? Does it feel ready to get this from my touch now? Are there any Parts not OK with this?"

- "What do you notice is happening with this place as you feel my touch? Are there any sensations anywhere else in your body? Are there any thoughts or feelings you are having?"

- "I am noticing _____ through my hand. Are you feeling this too?"

- "How are you feeling towards this Part I am touching? Would you like to convey that feeling yourself to this Part through your touch?"

When to Touch, When Not to Touch

When considering this question, the therapist starts with themselves. They work with their Parts to resolve their touch burdens. They unburden Parts with touch wounds—Parts that avoid touch, feel inadequate about touch, are desperate for touch, or lack appropriate boundaries. Supported by the practices of awareness, breath, resonance, and movement, connected with the Self Field, informed by professional ethical guidelines,[5] and receiving training and supervision in Attuned Touch, the therapist's touch can tacitly convey their Embodied Self energy.

The therapist considers many aspects of the client in determining whether their touch is appropriate. The client's touch history may include anything on a continuum from extreme neglect to extreme violations, such as physical abuse, physical assault, combat, sexual abuse, serious accidents, and medical procedures. Extreme touch wounds require a high degree of sensitivity. Touch or the prospect of touch may cause Parts to feel trapped, terrified, isolated, ashamed, sexually stimulated, numbed out, and confused as they are unable to discern safe and unsafe touch. Touch may be retraumatizing for the client's system. Traumatized Parts may result in the clients being over- or underresponsive to touch. The client's touch boundaries may be affected. Polarized Parts may oscillate between seeking inappropriate or unsafe touch and avoiding touch. Touch may be contraindicated with some trauma survivors until their system is healed enough to benefit from the healing power of touch.

The therapist considers the relational field with each client, aware that touch is filled with many layers of meaning, both psychological and cultural. The sexual, touch, and trauma history of the client and therapist, the culture and religion of the client and therapist, and the gendered or hierarchical nature of the therapist-client relationship are some of the layers that are considered. The therapist considers the client's stage in their healing process, and the level of safety established in their therapeutic relationship.

As many times as needed, the therapist communicates to the client about the safe boundaries, and that the client is in charge of the touch. The therapist relies on the practices of Somatic IFS to read and respond to the client's verbal and nonverbal somatosensory messages through touch so that they can sensitively track the client's nonverbal responses to the touch within their own body and the client's.

The therapist considers themselves, the client, and the therapeutic relationship to determine the appropriateness of Attuned Touch. They may assess that touch may not be appropriate for some clients, even if they ask for it. Touch may not be appropriate for some therapists, or with some or all of their clients. The assessment of when to use or not use this powerful practice calls on the therapist's deepest Self-led judgment and wisdom.

THE THERAPIST

- Touch, sexual, and trauma history
- Ability to set boundaries
- Culture, religion, gender, race, ethnicity, nationality
- Professional regulations or ethical and legal guidelines that may prohibit touch

- Fears that touch will evoke romantic, sexual, or perpetrator transference
- Ability to read nonverbal messages regarding response to touch

THE CLIENT

- Touch, sexual, and trauma history
- Ability to access Parts
- Ability to access Self
- Ability to set boundaries
- Ability to distinguish between safe and unsafe touch
- Ability to receive touch without retraumatization
- Culture, religion, gender, race, ethnicity, nationality

THE THERAPEUTIC RELATIONSHIP

- Sufficient safety and trust
- Gendered or hierarchical nature of the relationship
- Clear boundaries around touch (not sexual)
- Permission from all Parts for touch

FURTHER CONSIDERATIONS FOR TOUCH BURDENS OF THERAPIST AND CLIENT

- Parts activated by physical contact
- Parts unresponsive (numbing, dissociating) or overresponsive to touch
- Parts that misperceive touch as abusive, sexual, invasive, or controlling
- Parts that desperately crave touch and seek inappropriate touch
- Touch boundaries that are rigid, loose, or diffused
- Compliant Parts that verbally agree to the suggestion or expectation of touch
- Parts that reenact their unresolved trauma, either perpetrating or casting the person touching as the perpetrator
- Parts that sexualize all touch
- Parts that reject and resist touch
- Polarized Parts regarding touch
- With both therapist and client with access to Embodied Self energy, and with permission from the client's Parts in charge of the touch, Attuned Touch can reveal and heal clients' stories of physical neglect and abusive touch encoded in sensations and frozen movement. Attuned Touch may provide the missing experience that Parts have longed for.

Integration of Attuned Touch

Whether the touch is imaginary, our self touch, or touch from a friend or a professional, Attuned Touch in Somatic IFS harnesses the healing potential and avoids the harm of this powerful nonverbal communication. Attuned Touch establishes and strengthens the relational attachment between Parts and Self. Even more than tone of voice, facial expression, or posture, touch tacitly conveys Self energy to a Part, repairing wounds of attachment emotionally, somatically, socially, relationally, and neurologically.

1. Did you find you were able to "listen" with your hand to the tissues it was making contact with? If so, what did you notice?

_____

_____

_____

2. Did you find any Parts through Attuned Touch that you didn't know before, or know more deeply now? How did this Part respond to the touch?

_____

_____

_____

3. Were you able to help a Part repair its wounds of touch?

_____

_____

_____

4. Did you find Parts that need the support and guidance of a therapist to release its touch burdens?

_____

_____

_____

5. What do your Parts need in the future to integrate, reinforce, or anchor any shifts in your system?

_____

_____

_____

6. Did anything surprise you? Confuse you?

_____

_____

_____

7. If you are a therapist, what are some of the main takeaways from this chapter?

_____

_____

_____

Notes

1 Susan McConnell, *Somatic Internal Family Systems Therapy,* 219.

2 Susan McConnell, *Somatic Internal Family Systems Therapy,* 217–18.

3 Susan McConnell, *Somatic Internal Family Systems Therapy,* 243.

4 Susan McConnell, *Somatic Internal Family Systems Therapy,* 236.

5 See the US Association of Body Psychotherapy Code of Ethics, pp. 245–46, https://usabp.org/USABP-Code -of-Ethics.

7

The Internal Family Embodied

In the body we find it all. The burdens are in the body, the original gifts are in the body, and the qualities of Self energy are in the body. The most holy qualities of our Parts and Self buried deep in our body are a source of wisdom, strength, and healing. With Self energy in its embodied state through the practices of Somatic IFS, our buried resources are discovered, excavated, and reinstated. Our Parts are freed from the roles forced upon them and can resume or assume harmonious, collaborative roles and relationships with each other and with Self. Their functions, their tasks, and their characters emerge in ways and times appropriate to the current situation. Our inheritance is restored.[1]

SOMATIC IFS PRACTICES—by embodying Parts in our internal systems so they can be found, fully witnessed, and unburdened—lead to the liberation and embodiment of Self energy, individually and societally. We find Self energy in every Part, cell, and structure of the body. When in this state, unencumbered by our burdened Parts, we are freed to live out a harmonious relationship with our bodies, other human beings, and all living beings.

The previous chapters explored the individual and clinical applications of the five practices with the goal of Embodied Self. *Self energy* as well as *embodiment* can seem to elude definition. In my book, I suggest the following definition of *embodiment*:

> The subjective experience of being in our body, being present to our moment-by-moment sensations and movement impulses. More fundamentally embodiment could be described as *being* bodies, as *being* our sensations and movements.[2]

As you have learned, Self is often described by the qualities one experiences when in this state, many of which begin with the letter *C*—clarity, curiosity, courage, compassion, confidence, creativity, calmness, and connectedness. These qualities are inherent, embodied states. With this next exercise, you can experience these qualities through each of the five somatic practices to anchor them in your bodymind system.

EXPERIENTIAL EXERCISE
EMBODYING QUALITIES OF SELF

1. Choose one of the qualities of Self you want to experience in your body. It might be one of the *C* words (clarity, curiosity, courage, compassion, confidence, creativity, calmness, connectedness), or it might be presence, openness, acceptance, or other words that fit for you. If any Parts come up during this exercise, notice them and ask them to relax for now.

2. Invite that quality of Self energy to be expressed in your body. Where in your body do you feel it? What is the size, the shape? Where are the edges of it? What is the weight, the texture? Does this place have a color?

3. Are there sensations that go with this quality? If so, stay with them and invite them to sequence through your body. See if they want to become amplified.

4. Does your breathing change in any way?

5. Can you express this quality through movement? Let the movement unfold.

6. Does this place in your body where you feel Self energy want touch, or do you want to express this energy through touch?

7. Are there words or sounds that go with this quality?

8. Have these somatic practices made any shifts in this quality of Self? What worked best for you to support and anchor this quality?

9. Choose another quality of Self and bring each of the five practices to this quality.

Clinical Application of Somatic IFS

The publication of *Somatic Internal Family Systems Therapy* in 2020 has touched many more people than I could have imagined. To address the needs of many therapists, practitioners, and clients, my staff has grown and bloomed. Without their enthusiasm, support, and commitment, and without the enthusiasm of my readers and those eager to experience my Somatic IFS programs, I and this body of work might have benignly faded away into some version of semiretirement. Instead, Somatic IFS continues to grow and evolve because of this staff and our participants. I am proud to share their expertise with you.

Considerations:

- The experienced Somatic IFS staff members, clients, and program participants included in this chapter and throughout the workbook have generously submitted descriptions of their sessions and experiences using some or all of the five somatic practices integrated with the IFS Model.

- Various clinical issues will be mentioned.

SAFETY GUIDELINES

If you experience Parts being activated while reading any case example, the Somatic IFS practices can be a resource to bring Embodied Self to the burdened Parts.

- Some SIFS staff describe several sessions with one client, while others share one session applying one or two of the SIFS practices to various clinical issues.
  - For instance, the first example portrays several sessions with the same client, demonstrating how the practices assist with every step of the IFS Model. It is also a demonstration that Somatic IFS does not require the therapist to use words like *Part, Self, exile, manager,* or *firefighter,* but attunes to the verbal and nonverbal communication of the client.
- With deep gratitude for my staff, their clients, and the participants in my Somatic IFS retreats and trainings for helping Somatic IFS evolve, I share these clinical examples with you.
- The first example portrays several sessions with the same client demonstrating how the practices assist with every step of the model. It is also a demonstration that Somatic IFS does not require the therapist to use words like *Part, Self, exile, manager,* or *firefighter* but attunes to the verbal and nonverbal communication of the client.

SIFS with Weight Stigma and Body Shame
SIFS STAFF: MARCELLA COX
CLIENT: ROSE

Rose is a forty-three-year-old White, married, cisgender mother of three sons and professor at a prestigious university in Silicon Valley. She has lived in a larger body her whole life. Rose has multiple chronic health conditions, including celiac disease, small intestinal bacterial overgrowth (SIBO), irritable bowel syndrome (IBS), and polycystic ovary syndrome (PCOS). She has experienced weight stigma and fat shaming throughout her life, including by medical professionals. She and I have been working together for more than five years. When we began working together, Rose was struggling with an obsession about healthy eating and increased fears and anxiety around food due to her many health conditions, and her anxiety was having a negative impact on the quality of her life.

Rose came to a recent session outraged, sharing about an interaction with a customer at the grocery store. Her in-laws were coming from out of town for a week-long visit during her children's spring break, and she went to the grocery store to prepare for their visit. While standing in line, the customer in front of her looked at her and then at her cart before shaking her head and making a disdainful "tsk, tsk" sound. My client did her best to ignore this customer's judgments. After Rose checked out, she walked to her car only to find that the customer in line with her was now nearby in the parking lot. As Rose walked past her, the customer made a fat shaming comment, telling her she should cut down on the amount that she eats. Once again, Rose ignored the comment, went home, and ended up binge-eating "healthy food."

Somatic Awareness with Unblending

When Rose came to our session, she was visibly upset about the interaction. After meeting her pain with my compassionate care for how she was hurt and speaking for a Part of me that was also angry at what had happened, I invited Rose to notice what was happening in her body. She felt tension and pent-up energy coursing through her entire body. I asked Rose if it was all right for us to be with it just as it was. This helped Rose slow down, which I noticed in her breathing. She said she wasn't aware of this tension and agitation before, and she was OK to be with it. I asked her if the tension and agitation could sense that she was feeling them. She said they now could. I asked if these sensations would like Rose to know more. She reported that the sensations were intensifying in her arms. When I asked how she felt towards the sensation, she said she felt curious.

Mindful Movement with a Protector

As Rose was attending to the tension and agitation in her arms, I asked her if there was a movement her arms wanted to make. Rose quickly pushed with her arms and quietly responded "no." I reflected back that Rose was pushing away with her arms and asked her how her arms felt. Rose responded that they didn't feel any different. I invited her to experiment with it and either move them slowly or quickly and be with her arms as they moved. Rose stood up, and she slowly and forcefully pushed with her arms—this time with open hands, as if pushing someone away. She also stated "no" firmly and clearly, and it seemed to come from a deeper place in her body. I checked in with her again, and she expressed feeling a lot of relief. There was initially a smile on her face, and I invited her to just breathe into that place that felt the relief.

Conscious Breathing and Radical Resonance to Witness the Nonverbal Story of an Exile

I began noticing an ache in my heart, and as I felt the ache, Rose's eyes began to well up with tears. She said she was feeling grief for all the times that people made mean, fat-shaming comments about her body and she couldn't do anything about it. I told her that her tears and grief were welcome, and that we have space for however it wants to be known. I asked if she would like to send her grief a breath from her to welcome it too. As she did, she began to cry. I reassured her grief that it made sense, and I encouraged Rose to let the grief know it was being felt by her by sending it her breath. Rose stated that sending the grief her breath was helpful because it was like "her breath was touching and caressing a very painful place in her heart."

Somatic Awareness with Unburdening of an Exile

As Rose's tears began to subside, I asked her if the grief or the painful place had more it wanted her to feel, sense, or know. She said yes, that she is with her eleven-year-old self who is about to be weighed at school with all of her classmates. Her younger self, who had just begun menstruating, sees that her body is bigger and taller than the other girls. I asked Rose if she was with her eleven-year-old, and Rose replied that she was but her younger self couldn't sense her. I asked Rose how she felt towards her, and Rose said she had so much compassion for her and how hard that experience was. I asked her where she felt that compassion in her body. She said it was in her front body, especially in her heart. I asked if it felt right to send some of that compassionate energy to her eleven-year-old. As she did, Rose shared that her younger self could sense Rose. She showed Rose how horrified she felt hearing the PE teacher call out everyone's weight for the whole class to hear after they stepped on the scale.

Rose said that her younger self asked Rose to be next to her because she was scared everyone would know that she was the heaviest person in the class. As Rose moved next to her, Rose said that she could sense how scared and angry her eleven-year-old self felt about everyone around her seeing her body as different from theirs. Rose spoke sweetly to her eleven-year-old and let her know her feelings made sense. She also saw her eleven-year-old self look longingly at the flat chests and skinny legs of the girls in her class. Rose said she could feel her humiliation and shame for having the body she had. I asked her how she sensed the humiliation and shame. She said it was an icky feeling, powerless to tell her PE teacher that she didn't want to be weighed, and she couldn't run away. There was nothing she could do to stop it.

I asked if a re-do of this moment felt right. I told her inside that she can do that. Rose's younger self was initially in disbelief, but was so happy to stand up to her PE teacher, push him away, and say "no," just like she did earlier in our session. Her younger self said the PE teacher could have her icky feeling and weigh that instead. She slowly and methodically wiped off the icky feeling that was covering her entire body. She said it was a big sticky ball, and she gave it to her PE teacher. She watched him lift the heavy ball of ickiness to weigh it and walked away with her dignity.

Attuned Touch with Integration and Completion Stages

Her younger self then wanted a hug. As Rose was hugging her, I asked Rose to notice what that embrace felt like to her younger self. She said she liked feeling the warmth of her arms around her. The embrace felt like it was caring for and protecting her and her dignity. I invited my client to breathe in that sense of being embraced with care and protection so that energy was embodied and to anchor that felt sense.

Somatic Awareness and Conscious Breathing
with Polarizations, Trauma, and Legacy Burdens
SIFS STAFF: SHERRY RUBIN
CLIENT: MARY

A successful academic, Mary told me she was comfortable living from "her head up." A history of sexual and medical trauma, as well as religious and cultural legacy burdens, had built a fortress around what her body had experienced and what her body desired and continues to desire. Mary named one protector "Dignity" to refer to upholding beliefs and behaviors that were "right and acceptable." This Part did not want her "Life-force and alive energy" Part to be expressed for fear that she could lose relationships and community. She had found polarized Parts.

Mary was invited to create welcoming space for both these Parts. I asked, "Are you aware of these Parts? Are they aware of you?" Life-force took on a life of its own, blended because it had been exiled for so long. Rather than focus on the Self-to-Part relationship, she invited the Part to fully show itself, by continuing to blend, so that Mary could know it better. Could she engage with the sensations, and let Life-force know she felt her? Her smile and relaxed posture told me that this was a good way to understand. After some moments of this, I asked if Mary was aware of the Part, and how she felt towards it, and thus began the Self-to-Part relationship.

After staying there awhile, I asked her to notice her breath, and if it felt right, to breathe space for her Life-force, naming the sensations to herself and flowing with them; Mary began to sway and a smile found its way across her face. I invited her to notice what this felt like in the front, back, and middle body . . . to acknowledge and honor this experience, promising to return in a few minutes, but now to turn her attention to Dignity. And here she practiced, listening to my prompts, getting to know, understand, and be with this energy of Dignity in much the same way she had with Life-force.

Dignity showed her images of her intention to keep Mary safe, keep her connected to her family and her community. Following my invitations, Mary toggled back and forth, becoming more and more silent as images and felt senses without words unfolded. Prompts helped Mary deepen into her experiences. "Who is aware of what is happening?" "How do you feel towards this Part?" "Can you show these Parts they are not alone, that you are there?"

My last request was for her to experience both Parts at the same time, a nondual invitation. Mary had an embodied experience of how there could be welcoming and spaciousness for polarized Parts, and a taste of possibility for the future.

Somatic Awareness for Witnessing the Unburdening of an Exile's Body Story for Intergenerational Healing
SIFS STAFF: SONIA MILOHANIC
CLIENT: OLIVER

This process extended over two sessions. Oliver described a sense of being "stuck" and "trapped" in his life and responsibilities. As he spoke, I invited him to notice any sensations in his body. He described a "big hole in his gut." He also noticed a heaviness in his shoulders and a sense of being "pushed down."

We attended to several concerned Parts with agendas to go fast and not to feel, and they agreed to give space while offering their intentions to support the healing process. As they unblended, Oliver was able to access some embodied Self energy, which he described as a tingling and thrumming in the rest of his body. He felt interested towards the hole in his belly. I invited him to offer this sense of thrumming interest directly to his belly.

Oliver sensed the Part needed darkness, so he turned off the light in his room. With Oliver's permission, I invited the Part to get bigger in his body so we could really witness its body story.

As he returned his awareness to the hole, he had a strong feeling of being trapped, scared, and unable to breathe. His face felt scrunched up and he noticed tears at the back of his eyes and feelings of deep sadness and aloneness. He felt intense pressure on the top of his head, his spine, and then everywhere, like his whole body was being crushed. He drew his head towards his belly.

I asked whether there were any images that went with these sensations, and he saw a fetus and images of being birthed. He felt pressure around his neck and had an image of the umbilical cord there. He felt the Part's fear, confusion, and loneliness.

Oliver then described bright light, unfamiliar voices, and sadness as the cord was cut and the Part felt it had "left being a Part of her," which was "like a death." He then experienced the warmth of his mother's skin and her touch as she cradled and comforted the Part. The Part felt pure love, joy, and relief. He could see the Part dancing as it experienced his Self presence through the birthing process, that it was no longer alone.

I was aware that Oliver's mother had died some years before, so I asked whether it felt right to invite her energy into the scene. He said it felt as though "a door had been opened" as his mother's spirit joined him and the infant Part, touching both of them, as well as other Parts in his system. Oliver later described it as "one of the most powerful experiences of my life."

Conscious Breathing and Attuned Touch with Legacy Burdens of Physical Symptoms
SIFS STAFF: SHERRY RUBIN AND HER CLIENT

My client came to her session with a headache. As the client wondered if the two-day headache could be connected with stress, they spontaneously put their hands on their forehead. I suggested they notice the sensations of the headache and the felt sense of the touch. The client shared feeling "jammed up with some Parts trying to ram through the clog." It felt like "very uncomfortable pushing, frenzied energy responding to all the things needing to be done." I gently invited my client to "just stay there and breathe, let the breath make space for it."

Their next comment was that it was related to their mother, and then a description of the mother that sounded like the energy they were experiencing in their head—an urgency of trying to figure it out, fix the jam, get things going. And after a few more minutes of being with it, observing, and sensing this energy, I asked what percentage of the energy was their mother's. "Almost all of it," they responded. I said, "See if the Parts know this is your mother's energy or if this is news to them." It was revelatory, completely novel news. The session ended with the client allowing this information to settle in, updating with the news that this was not their energy, and returning, reclaiming, and honoring their own way of dealing with challenges, not their mother's.

Radical Resonance with a Couple
SIFS STAFF: LADONNA SILVA AND HER CLIENTS

While I am working with a couple dealing with infidelity, my body resonates with that of the male partner who, being yelled at by his wife, shrinks in his chair. After taking a pause to help the female client's protectors regulate, I bring her awareness to the solid rock she feels in her stomach. Briefly tuning in to her stomach, she finds Parts with burdens of powerlessness and fear. Understanding this area is connected energetically with confidence and power, she brings her hand to this energy center, communicating reassurance to her Parts. She takes a deep breath and lets her Parts know she is available after the session to connect with them.

I refocus on the male client, and he finds the Part that was shrinking, trying to hide, get small, and escape. I ask if this Part is anywhere in his body. He does not find it in his body, but he shares a childhood memory of verbal and physical abuse. With successive sessions, I find that adjusting the seating to provide more physical space, slowing the session down, taking frequent pauses, and focusing on body and breathing bring more depth to the interactions and dynamics of the couple.

They come to understand they both have Parts that carry burdens of powerlessness, for different reasons with different responses. My resonance with their issues of powerlessness held by my embodied Self supports their continued work as my presence brings an open-hearted, resonant, balanced neutral presence to this couple navigating a challenging situation.

Mindful Movement with Polarized Parts
SIFS THERAPIST: JUDITH FISCHER
CLIENT: PATTI

Patti is aware of how she pushes people away, including me, and how it interferes with her current relationships. Her reaching-out Part polarizes with the pushing-away Part. Working virtually, I noticed Patti's hands and wrists move outwards when she spoke for the pushing-away Part and inwards when she spoke of wanting to take someone in. We explored these movements together, exaggerating them, playing with the pace and force, and adding the words that came to them with the movements. "Go away from me," "Please don't leave," "Don't come any closer," "Will you stay with me?" "I don't want you here," "I like playing with you," "This is ridiculous." Patti came to understand her pushing-away Part tries to protect the Part that believes she does not deserve to be loved. As the session came to a close, she came to the clarity that she could "pause and choose" when to receive and when to push away in relationships.

Mindful Movement and Attuned Touch with Complex PTSD
SIFS THERAPIST: JUDITH FISCHER
CLIENT: TOMMY

Tommy is a veteran Marine from the War in Afghanistan with complex PTSD. After working unsuccessfully with several therapists, telling the same stories over and over, he had been feeling increasingly helpless and suicidal and was appreciating Somatic IFS and movement with his sessions with me. As he shared his grief and loneliness about losing friends in the war and from suicide, I sat silently with him as we both held one hand on the back of our heads and the other hand on our hearts, gently rocking side to side. He said he no longer felt so alone in the minefields and dark forest. I suggested we move together through the minefields, stopping occasionally to breathe and to ground by rooting into the earth. He told me that moving between freezing with fear and holding his heart, with my presence, relieved his fear and locked up feeling.

Mindful Movement and Attuned Touch for Embryological, Multigenerational, and Racial Healing
SIFS RETREAT PARTICIPANT: ANA

During the movement practice, first I felt a need for quietness, almost no movement. That is significant for me because I have a "doer" Part that keeps me in constant motion. Then I felt a sense of being rocked. I remember La Loba (a female archetype from *Women Who Run with the Wolves* who sang over the bones, and then rocked that being back to life). I felt like my five-year-old Part and my in utero Part were gently rocked, over and over and over, by this gentle warm beautiful being (my Self? La Loba?).

As I was being rocked, I felt the presence of my mother, grandmother, and great grandmother on my left side also rocking me. Then the music changed to a more tribal tune, and I felt the presence of many beings surrounding us in a circle, with arms linked and moving gently, rocking us even more.

(A couple of years ago, during a meditation, I had experienced the presence of these same beings during the moment of my birth, and the death of my mother alone in a hospital due to COVID, telling us: "You are not alone; we are here with you; we are celebrating you.")

Then, I thought that even when I was in utero, my eggs were already there. So, I thought about bringing the presence of my two daughters, ages twenty-eight and twenty-one, to the circle. But also they have their eggs within them, so I brought the future generations to our healing circle. As we were all rocking gently together, I felt that all this rocking was not only for me, Ana. At that moment, the images became a bit fuzzy, the shapes were not so defined, and I felt like every being in the circle took turns coming in and out of the middle to experience being rocked by all the rest of the beings. What a sense of support and connection!

Then we were encouraged to go and share our experiences with others. Magically or spontaneously, the four BIPOC people from my small group came together, and we shared our stories. One of them talked about not being wanted by her mother, who attempted to terminate her life. That gave her the message "I am not supposed to be here," which has persisted throughout her life. The other two members also shared their own stories of pain and disconnection. I was reluctant to share my experience because it was so different from theirs. But after being asked to share, I realized that my experience was also for them to experience a sense of healing, connection, and support.

The day of Attuned Touch, I had the opportunity to share with the same participant who experienced the rejection of her mother in the womb. Together, we created an image of each of us being in a very warm, nurturing womb, with amniotic fluid surrounding us filled with love, strength, and the power to protect us from any harm and keep us safe so that we can become!

Finally, at the last dinner together, I witnessed the powerful connection Susan had with another participant. My heart melted under the presence of so much love, healing, connection, and repair work that happened. Two generations coming together, two races coming together in a beautiful repairing, healing moment.

Attuned Touch with Complex Trauma
SIFS STAFF: LADONNA SILVA
CLIENT: CW

I use Attuned Touch with my client "CW," who has dissociative identity disorder and complex trauma, to help them (CW's pronouns are *they* and *them*) physically experience Self energy. CW's breath is shallow, their eyes darting around the room. Their four-year-old Part is in great despair and fear, desperate to connect with a safe adult. CW and I sit together on the ground. CW asks to be cuddled like a baby. I check in with CW's protectors, who have come to trust me, and they are OK with this physical intimacy for a short time. I also check in with my own system. My heart softens, I breathe more deeply, and I rest into my calm center. I shift my position to be able to support this touch. I slow down the process and track for activation as CW rests their head on my legs while lying on the ground curled up. When I notice CW squirming and tightening, I ask again if the physical connection is OK with their Parts. CW's body softens as their four-year-old Part receives this needed parent-like protection until they can find their own Self energy. I softly hold my hand on CW's head.

Attuned Self Touch with Sexuality and Intergenerational Burdens
SIFS STAFF: KARBY ALLINGTON-GOLDFAIN
CLIENT: KATIE

Katie began the session sitting in her garage and stating she needed to stretch as we talked as she didn't feel present in her body. Her request for the session was for help being more present with her partner during sexual interactions. Katie expressed that she wasn't sure what she even needed or what to request from her partner.

As I was curious about the Parts of her that dissociate or distance during sexual interactions, I noticed Katie rubbing her hip. I paused and asked Katie to check and ask if her hip needed or wanted some attention. Katie took her awareness into her body and said she immediately heard "yes." As we were curious, her body brought awareness that there was a line of connection from her hip to her brain and then a branch of that connection that included her heart.

We held space and opened to that awareness and connection. As the connection opened and energy was flowing from hip to heart and brain, the hip brought an image of black gunk that it was holding. Katie felt curious about this, as did I, and as she listened, she heard that most of it came from her family of origin, but a strand came from another relative who was coming to visit soon. Katie also noticed the presence of Self energy below the area of gunk in her hip. As we were aware of and curious about the hip, Katie continued to hold her hip with her hand and her hip communicated it felt support and connection through Katie's hand.

We asked the hip if it felt it needed to continue to hold this strand of black gunk. The hip let us know it was ready to release it. Katie verbalized the return of the black strand to the relative to whom it belonged and felt it go out of her hip. She spontaneously spoke of the need for discernment during the upcoming visit on how to be kind without taking on any of this person's energy and her confidence that Self could provide this discernment.

Katie's countenance visibly softened and opened as she reported the difference in her whole body and the sense of being present inside her own body.

With some time left in the session, I asked Katie if she still had interest in her original question about being present with her partner during sexual interactions. Katie laughed and shared that she had already made the connection in her mind. Katie stated with clarity that something she needs from her partner is for him to hold space for her in some areas of life where she is making some significant decisions. For her to feel he is holding her struggle without providing a solution. Katie felt she could explore with her partner how that could be accomplished without taking on the burden of figuring it all out ahead of time and telling him exactly how to support her. We explored how this shift in the dynamic could have a direct impact on their sexual interactions and Katie's capacity to feel deeply connected and present.

Attuned Touch with Attachment Wounds
CLIENT: STEF COLEMAN, MFT, A CLIENT OF SOMATIC IFS STAFF BETH ONEIL

I came into the session aching, lonely, sad, feeling isolated. I don't fit in, nothing ever feels quite right, I'm all alone.

Thankfully I have a very deep trust and connection with my IFS therapist I was blessed to work with and build a relationship in person at a Somatic IFS retreat in Hawaii, now two years ago. I have been working with this therapist about once a month in these past two years.

Right away, when we came together on Zoom, I felt that I wanted to lay my head on her lap. So I decided to go with that. The desire was so strong I just went with it. What came to me in those moments was that IFS work is so imaginal anyway, I'm going to take this even farther and use my imagination through Zoom with my therapist.

So, as I knew she would, she welcomed me to go with my imagination, and she met me there. She said, "Yes, of course, lay your head down on my lap." I read in her face that the invitation was real. I closed my eyes as I sat upright in my chair facing the Zoom screen. Almost immediately, what I call Guidance, or Self, Pure Knowing, zinged in. I wanted and needed actual physical support. So, I got up and grabbed the long cushion from my couch that was nearby. I placed it lengthwise on my lap so that I could support my head leaning forward and resting on the end of it. It also felt great on my chest to have the support of the whole couch cushion. I was really supported on my head, enough to fully surrender to it. And I could feel the full contact with the cushion on my body, and I could surrender there as well.

I was still imagining my therapist supporting me, that it was her who was holding me. No matter what I needed to feel supported and held, it was my therapist accommodating me, attuning to me, unconditionally being with me in this support. Then I said, "Now you are holding my face with your warm loving hands," and I had a complete and total surrender. The surrender I felt was deep in my chest and heart and shoulders. Melting tears came easily and flowed down my face.

After about five or seven minutes (I process really quickly), I knew I had to lie down for much more support, so I went to the couch. I brought the laptop and put it on the coffee table, without leaving the deep space that was happening, and my therapist followed without a hitch. I made sure she could see me for the witnessing. It all went very smoothly. I lay down on the couch face up and closed my eyes once again. Having my therapist there on the computer was deeply impactful and was a huge part of me being able to drop in even more deeply.

Now I can really settle in, but I'm cold. I know I don't want more disruption, so instead of getting up for a blanket, I use the pillows on the couch. This ends up being delightful and very warm and cozy.

The melting and deepening is profound now. And my baby arrives. The baby me trapped in a crib all by herself, for hours at a time. She/I feel hopeless, helpless, sad, despondent. At this point the therapist asks how I feel towards the baby (Self to Part). A really sweet unblending happens there and quite quickly. I stay with the connection between me and the baby.

I am very comfortable lying there. I bend my knees and put a nice big pillow under them for support. I am feeling an all-encompassing holding, and goodness, real and true goodness. All the while the therapist is building Self-to-Part and Part-to-Self connection. I hear the therapist and I respond effortlessly. My primary response is one of deep relaxation with every breath. I cry, close to sobbing, relaxing, gently releasing. Crying has not come easily to me in the past.

I'm realizing how many Parts constellated and formed in me even so young! Hopeless Part, Trapped Part, Frozen Part, Confused Part, just to name a few. Even young, I started to turn on myself: "What's wrong with me that I can be left here all by myself?" I so yearn to be held, comforted, feel contact, to feel loved, and nothing. It does not make sense. It does not compute.

The therapist asks if the Part would like to leave that time (Retrieval) and she says, "Yes, please!" So we find the baby in her crib, and we've got here-and-now me, and I go to the crib to get her. Just being with her, her feeling me, and me feeling her, is everything. So much makes sense. It comes to me why I use alcohol. The lack of holding and contact and connection gets filled almost immediately with alcohol, or so it seems.

Something quite magical happens when baby and adult connect. A melting, a softening, a sense of "all is all right now." A settling, a sweetness, an internal bonding, some kind of palpable rewiring or something like that. Even in this moment of recounting all this, it is happening right now. She is a very happy baby. And my adult me is at peace as well.

A huge part of all of this is also the awareness of my managers, how busy and all-consuming with running my life they have been. I have been in a kind of survival my whole life, frantically on varying levels, to take care of the onslaught of life.

I have been working on myself for over thirty years. I was never aware of how run by my managers my whole life has been. I now see how "Busy" protects my vulnerable baby. These precious managers working so hard to protect the vulnerable baby. The baby feels so loved! She feels deeply loved maybe even for the first time in her life.

Everybody is in Meeting Place sitting around a roaring bonfire: warm and peaceful. The fire is burning bright and big. I have always loved fires. I can feel that it is a Source for me. All of my Parts are hanging out with each other. Some are mature, quiet, and peaceful—just relaxed. Some are young, innocent, playful, and sweet. There is a sense of togetherness.

With my therapist, I made a 100 percent promise to stay connected to my little one, and oh, she is so precious. She started out a skinny red baby. Now she is plump, and fleshy, and happy, smiley, giggly, and content.

Unburdening a Newborn Part with Somatic IFS

SIFS STAFF: ELLEN GROSSMAN

CLIENT: INDIE

Indie came to me for help integrating a ketamine-assisted therapy session in which she experienced being on the edge of a void, all alone and terrified that she would be sucked in and never return. Indie shared with me about her early attachment trauma. As a newborn, a blocked esophagus resulted in three weeks of extreme eating difficulties, followed by traumatic surgery to repair the esophagus, and then eight weeks of hospitalization and isolation in the NICU.

In the session, Indie described physical sensations that made no sense to her. "It feels like my entire torso is a void. There's no body there—no torso. Just arms, legs, and head put on an empty space. It feels like a big empty ball." She found a very young Part, hunched over, wearing a cloak that was protecting an egg of emptiness. "I see faces above me, but I feel *alone*. I don't matter. My needs don't matter. I'm *exposed*. No one will touch me, clean me. I have no skin. There's no one there to help me. It's up to me. If I don't scream, I'll be sucked into the void."

This Part asks Indie to put her hand under her bum to keep her from falling into the void. She wants eye contact with Indie to know that Indie is *here*, not up and out there. She says, "Don't let go of me." Indie takes this exile in her arms. "I gotcha," she says as she holds her and looks into her eyes.

Somatic IFS Practices with an Exile Part
SIFS STAFF: SONIA MILOHANIC
CLIENT: JENNY

Jenny had Parts ashamed and disgusted about her "neediness" and "greediness," particularly in her sexual relationship with her partner, Tim. As these Parts separated, Jenny's infant exile emerged, first as an image of a little one with its arms raised, desperately reaching out, and then with the words "help me, help me" and a sense of insatiable hunger and yearning.

I noticed Jenny's jaw slightly moving, and I invited Jenny to bring her awareness to her jaw. As she stayed with the sensations, Jenny felt a tingling in her mouth and a deep desire to suck. She heard the word "mine" and realized the Part wanted to drink milk from its mother's breast.

A Part reacted with disgust to the exile's desire to suckle the mother's breast, calling her mother a "villain witch" and the suckling a shameful sexual act. I suggested the infant Part could instead drink from Self's breast, not her mother's. The disgusted Part was OK with that.

Jenny turned off her camera and brought the infant Part to her chest. Jenny and the infant Part looked into each other's eyes. Jenny soothingly told the infant as she drank: "It's OK. It's OK. This is yours. It's OK to want. It's OK to need."

Somatically Anchoring an Unburdened Part
SIFS STAFF: SONIA MILOHANIC
CLIENT: PENNY

Penny was preparing to see her mother, with whom she had a tumultuous relationship. As we checked in with several young Parts, Penny noticed the posture of a recently unburdened Part. She saw the Part standing strong, not prepared to allow her mother's emotions to swallow her own.

I invited Penny to embody the posture, breathing it into her cells, fleshing it out. She described a grounded strength in her legs and felt herself growing taller, embodying a sense of dignity. Penny noticed her exhale lengthened as she stayed with this posture. As she exhaled, she noticed the breath creating a bubble-like force field extending about half a meter around her whole body. Inside the protection of the force field she felt a lightness and calm in her body. Penny agreed to revisit this experience between sessions and prior to meeting with her mother.

Integration of Somatic IFS

With a focus on the subjective, nonverbal, embodied expression of our internal and sociocultural systems, Somatic IFS humbly and gratefully embraces and participates in an emerging paradigm that challenges the four-hundred-year tradition of dualistic hierarchies at the core of Western social institutions, including psychology. As we embody our internal systems, Somatic IFS provides a path to unburden our cultural legacies of a passive, objectifying, and oppressive relationship with our bodies, others, and the earth. As we restore the original qualities to our Parts, we are free to live a more fully awakened, Self-led life.

We have experienced the many ways somatic practices, combined with the IFS Model, bring both nonverbal and verbal interventions to our individual and societal burdens. The practice of Somatic Awareness has helped us find our Parts and forge a compassionate relationship with them. As the Parts' body stories are witnessed, the sensations are invited to sequence through the body, releasing the physical, emotional, and behavioral burdens. Our Parts' essential nature is restored. Our senses are awakened. Our cells, organs, and tissues pulsate, collaborate, and communicate.

Our awareness flows between us and the world as we bring our conscious presence to our breathing. Our breath leads us to Parts who restrict our breathing, and we also discover that a few breaths can propel our system from its preoccupation with the past or the future, and into the present moment brimming with Self energy. Our breathing dissolves the boundaries of mind, body, and spirit, of internal and external, self and other.

The qualities of Self energy glide on the wings of our breath as we dive into the deep waters of a resonant relationship. Our heartfelt, radically resonant receptivity revises and repairs our body-based attachment wounds, rewiring both brain and body. The exponentially amplified frequencies of our resonant bodies are transmitted to every level of system, from the subatomic to the cosmic.

As we travel along the space-time continuum from conception to the present, we mindfully revisit our earliest developmental movements. We reconnect with the inherent life force of our primitively organized cells to attach, nourish, and protect. We explore and unburden our Parts' movement patterns acquired from developmental or ancestral traumas. Bringing mindfulness to our inherent adaptive responses to trauma, we slowly and safely revisit the Parts buried in our autonomic and neuromuscular systems. As the frozen or interrupted movement story sequences through the body, our Self energy is freely expressed in every move we make.

The practices of awareness, breath, resonance, and movement provide a foundation for incorporating what may be the most potent and effective form of nonverbal implicit communication between Parts and Self: touch. The tactile experience of safe, respectful, Attuned Touch is tacitly conveyed as Embodied Self energy travels along the skin, fascia, muscles, and nerves, unleashing a stream of healing chemicals and Self presence so desperately needed by Parts embedded in the tissues. In an increasingly virtual world in an already touch-deprived culture where physical and sexual abuse is rampant, the emancipation of ethical, appropriate touch from the shadows of fear and shame has the potential to transform social isolation, sensory deprivation, and wounds of touch both interpersonal and societal.

Somatic IFS is indebted to the IFS Model, to Richard Schwartz, and to all those whose contributions shaped and continue to shape the IFS Model. It also owes deep gratitude to the many leaders, teachers, and researchers who have developed the vast field of somatics and somatic psychotherapy over many decades, most notably Hakomi psychotherapy, but also sensorimotor therapy, Somatic Experiencing, Continuum Movement, and Body-Mind Centering.

With a mixture of gratitude and nostalgia, I continually bow to those teachers who were physically present with me over the years, whose presence and wisdom have informed and formed me and Somatic IFS. Their impact spans the fields of psychology, embodiment, and spirituality. Dick Schwartz, Jon Eisman, Ron Kurtz, Amina Knowlan, David Patterson, Bobby Rhodes, Susan Harper, Susan Aposhyan, Lisa Clark, Bonnie Bainbridge Cohen, Alan Davidson, Althea Orr, Ed Spencer, David Lauterstein, Vickie Dodd, Pat Ogden, Kekuni Minton, and Maura Sills. Many others have taught and influenced Somatic IFS through their writings and, more recently, online trainings, including Thomas Hübl, Fatimah Finney, and Resmaa Menakem. I am especially indebted to countless colleagues, friends, clients, staff, and graduates and participants of Somatic IFS programs who have supported, challenged, and contributed to Somatic IFS.

Notes

1 Susan McConnell, *Somatic Internal Family Systems Therapy,* 256–57.
2 Susan McConnell, *Somatic Internal Family Systems Therapy,* 255–56.

Resources

Visit my website, www.embodiedself.net, to sign up for my newsletter to find out about upcoming Somatic IFS programs. In addition to this newsletter, you can stay connected in the SIFS community by joining the Somatic IFS Google group at https://groups.google.com/g/somatic-ifs and the Somatic IFS group on Facebook: www.facebook.com/groups/6540285286076082.

Bibliography

Anderson, Frank G. *Transcending Trauma: Healing Complex PTSD with Internal Family Systems.* Eau Claire, WI: PESI, 2021.

Angelou, Maya. *I Shall Not Be Moved.* New York: Random House, 1991.

Aposhyan, Susan M. *Heart Open, Body Awake: Four Steps to Embodied Spirituality.* Boulder, CO: Shambhala, 2021.

Dana, Deb, and Courtney Rolfe. *Polyvagal Prompts: Finding Connection and Joy through Guided Explorations.* New York: W. W. Norton, 2024.

Eigen, Charles, ed. *Inner Dialogue in Daily Life: Contemporary Approaches to Personal and Professional Development in Psychotherapy.* London: Jessica Kingsley, 2014.

Hardy, Kenneth V. *The Enduring, Invisible, and Ubiquitous Centrality of Whiteness.* New York: W. W. Norton, 2022.

Hübl, Thomas. *Attuned: Practicing Interdependence to Heal Our Trauma—and Our World.* Boulder, CO: Sounds True, 2023.

Kopald, Seth. *Self-Led: Living a Connected Life with Yourself and with Others.* Ann Arbor, MI: Exploration Services, 2023.

Mate, Gabor. *The Myth of Normal: Trauma, Illness, & Healing in a Toxic Culture.* New York: Avery, 2022.

McConnell, Susan. *Somatic Internal Family Systems Therapy: Awareness, Breath, Resonance, Movement and Touch in Practice.* Berkeley, CA: North Atlantic Books, 2020.

Mischke-Reeds, Manuela. *Somatic Psychotherapy Toolbox: 125 Worksheets and Exercises to Treat Trauma & Stress.* Eau Claire, WI: PESI, 2018.

Porges, Stephen W. *The Polyvagal Theory: Neurophysiological Foundations of Emotions, Attachment, Communication, and Self-Regulation.* New York: W. W. Norton, 2011.

Riemersma, Jenna, ed. *Altogether Us: Integrating the IFS Model with Key Modalities, Communities, and Friends.* La Vergne, TN: Pivotal Press, 2023.

Schwartz, Richard C. *No Bad Parts: Healing Trauma and Restoring Wholeness with the Internal Family Systems Model.* Boulder, CO: Sounds True, 2021.

Sweezy, Martha. *Internal Family Systems Therapy for Shame and Guilt.* New York: Guilford Press, 2023.

Sweezy, Martha, and Ellen L. Ziskind. *Internal Family Systems Therapy: New Dimensions.* London: Routledge, 2013.

Acknowledgments

WITHOUT THE PUBLISHING TEAM at North Atlantic Books who saw the potential of this workbook and encouraged me to find the time to create it, this workbook would not exist. It was improved by Isabelle Felix's expert editing that brought clarity and structure while her enthusiasm, perspective, and marvelous smile and laugh warmed my heart. For me, writing is a largely solo endeavor, but I welcomed SIFS staff member Beth Rogerson's offer to review some of my earlier drafts.

Somatic IFS is the culmination of the wisdom, guidance, and inspiration of many teachers and leaders in the fields of psychotherapy and embodiment. Dick Schwartz receives my deep and lasting love and appreciation, along with Kay Gardner, who has journeyed with me from Hakomi to IFS and beyond. IFS Trainer friends and colleagues, clients and students, Hakomi trainers and students, many bodywork and movement teachers, and teachers of other clinical modalities have shaped my body and my body of work. I am grateful to Bobby Rhodes, a.k.a. Soeng Hyang, of the Kwan Um School of Zen Buddhism, for her foundational teachings.

The Somatic IFS retreats and trainings would not be possible without my beloved training staff, who, as of this writing, include Beth ONeil, Marcella Cox, Karby Allington-Goldfain, Maritza Erazu, LaDonna Silva, Nancy Berkowitz, Trish Attia, Dario Martinez, Sherry Rubin, Lesley Hartman, Irina Diyankova, Beth Rogerson, Sonia Milohanic, Christine Bombosch, Ellen Grossman, and Jo Chan. Many of them have contributed their thoughts and their case examples to this workbook. This international network of experienced, diverse staff continues to expand as they mentor Somatic IFS therapists to assist in programs where they facilitate participants' embodiment of their internal systems and supervise practice groups. They offer therapy and consultation and, in countless ways, enrich and extend the reach and ripple effect of Somatic IFS. I am grateful for their solid commitment, wisdom, and support.

My most dedicated staff member, Beth ONeil, has a far more important role in my life. Without this woman as my life partner and wife, I would not be who I am today. It would take another book to convey the depth of my love and gratitude for all that we have shared over forty years—from building a home, raising a daughter, traveling to teach IFS and Somatic IFS, and now enjoying our grandchildren. Impressively, as I abandon her to write, teach, and tend to business, she does everything else to maintain our home and social life, while still joining and supporting me in all my endeavors. And she mostly stays in Embodied Self the entire time.

My heartfelt gratitude goes to all those worldwide who have read my book *Somatic Internal Family Systems Therapy*. My sincere hope is that this workbook will deepen your understanding towards restoring Embodied Self energy.

About the Author

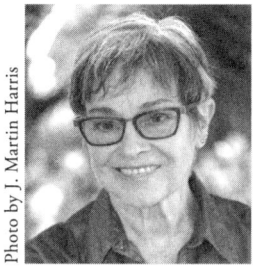

Photo by J. Martin Harris

Susan McConnell, MAPD, CHT, somatic therapist, educator, developer, and author, has been passionately committed to restoring the holism of body and mind in healing individual and societal wounds. The intersection of body and mind was the foundation of all her professional experiences—from directing the counseling program at Chicago's first domestic violence shelter, integrating psychotherapy and bodywork in her treatment of trauma survivors, founding and directing a group practice for psychotherapists and bodyworkers, and culminating in thirty years of a body-centered approach in her teaching of Hakomi and IFS to therapists and practitioners.

Susan was drawn to the IFS Model in the mid-1990s for its nonpathologizing, empowering approach to personal and systemic transformation. She soon became a Senior Lead Trainer for the IFS Institute, where she was instrumental in designing training programs, developing curricula, mentoring trainers, and bringing the IFS model to the world for which she received the first Lifetime Achievement Award.

Somatic IFS has been woven by these many threads, as well as by Susan's Zen Buddhist and earth-based spiritual practices, various movement modalities, and social activism. Somatic IFS workshops, retreats, and trainings bring embodiment to the internal family by applying somatic practices to IFS therapy. Susan continues to be inspired by the potential of a somatic approach to therapy to liberate our true essential Selves and to dismantle the culture's mind-body hierarchical dualism embedded in our bodies and our institutions.

Susan is the author of *Somatic Internal Family Systems Therapy: Awareness, Breath, Resonance, Movement and Touch in Practice* (2020) as well as chapters in *Altogether Us: Integrating the IFS Model with Key Modalities, Communities, and Friends,* edited by Jenna Riemersma (2023); *Internal Family Systems Therapy: New Dimensions,* edited by Martha Sweezy and Ellen L. Ziskind (2013); and *Inner Dialogue in Daily Life: Contemporary Approaches to Personal and Professional Development in Psychotherapy,* edited by Charles Eigen (2014).

About North Atlantic Books

North Atlantic Books (NAB) is an independent, nonprofit publisher committed to a bold exploration of the relationships between mind, body, spirit, and nature. Founded in 1974, NAB aims to nurture a holistic view of the arts, sciences, humanities, and healing. To make a donation or to learn more about our books, authors, events, and newsletter, please visit www.northatlanticbooks.com.